Praying
Through Your
Pregnancy

Regal

From Gospel Light
Ventura, California, U.S.A.

Published by Regal
From Gospel Light
Ventura, California, U.S.A.
www.regalbooks.com
Printed in the U.S.A.

Library of Congress Cataloging-in-Publication Data
Polimino, Jennifer.
Praying through your pregnancy : an inspirational week-by-week guide
for moms-to-be/ Jennifer Polimino, Carolyn Warren.
p. cm.
ISBN 978-0-8307-4808-2 (hardcover)
1. Pregnant women—Prayers and devotions. 2. Christian women—Prayers
and devotions. I. Warren, Carolyn. II. Title.
BV4847.P66 2010
242'.6431—dc22
2009050689

Rights for publishing this book outside the U.S.A. or in non-English languages are administered by Gospel Light Worldwide, an international not-for-profit ministry. For additional information, please visit www.glww.org, email info@glww.org, or write to Gospel Light Worldwide, 1957 Eastman Avenue, Ventura, CA 93003, U.S.A.

Dedication

Jennifer Polimino:
For my children, Micah Kekoa and Malia Grace.
Without you, this book would not be.
I love you both more than you'll ever know.

Carolyn Warren:
For my children, Ryan and Wendy.
You have brought me joy and gladness.

Contents

Part IV: Third Trimester
(WEEKS 28 TO BIRTH)

Appendices: Something More

Acknowledgments

We give honor to our mothers, Sharon Joy and Barbara Jean, two beautiful women who taught us the power of prayer.

A big thank-you to our literary agent, John Willig, president of Literary Services, Inc., for believing in our message and our ability to express it on the written page. We appreciate the counsel he gave us along the way to help make this project a success.

Heartfelt appreciation goes to Steven Lawson, for his vision and expertise in shepherding our project from start to finish. Thank you to Mark Weising for his proficient supervision of the copyediting stage, and to the entire team at Regal Books in Ventura, California.

We want to thank the courageous women who shared their beautiful pregnancy and birth stories with us: Kimberly Grano, Karen Johnson and her daughter Haley Tizzard, Jo Lembo and her daughter Betsy Leeuwner, Holly Montoya, Nancy Rice, Barb Rickford and Darla Sanborn. Also, a special thank-you to Janet Grabe, Jennifer's doula extraordinaire, for her support and help in recording both of her birth stories; and to Betty Fire, Jennifer's dear friend and favorite massage therapist, for helping her during her pregnancies.

We express our gratitude to Debbie Mills, Prayer Leader for Prenatal Prayer at the International House of Prayer (IHOP), for sharing her spiritual insight and testimonies with us. And our respect goes to Director Mike Bickle for being the pioneer who started IHOP.

We thank our church pastors—Pastor Blake LaMunyon at Cherry Hills Community Church in Colorado, Pastor Gordon Banks at New Heart Worship Center, and Pastor Joe Turner at Shorewood Foursquare Church in Washington—for their teaching on faith and prayer and for watching over our souls.

Love from Jennifer to Dan, and from Carolyn to Brandon, our husbands who gave us their support and encouragement.

And most of all, we thank and give praise to Jesus Christ, our Lord and Savior. We give the credit to Him for the idea for this book; for the ability and stamina to write it in less than three months; and for making it possible for us to meet up with each other—across the States via the Internet—in the first place.

PART I

Conception

(WEEKS 1 AND 2)

I chose you before I formed you in the womb;
I set you apart before you were born.
JEREMIAH 1:5

1

God's Timing for Your Baby

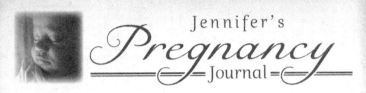

Jennifer's
Pregnancy
Journal

It's been over four months of "trying" and we're still not pregnant. I'm not sure what is going on.

Maybe we are too old—I'm 35 and Dan is 37. Did we wait too long?

We've been married more than five years, and I've been the one who wanted to wait, and now I'm secretly crying every month when I get my period.

I was at lunch the other day with two of my girlfriends, and I broke down again over the fact that we're still not pregnant! They both have children, so I don't think they truly understand.

Maybe God doesn't think I'll be a good mother. There were many times in my life when I said, "I will never have kids." Maybe God heard me and listened.

But in my heart, I know that's not true. I know I just need to wait upon God. He knows when I'm ready.

I've been praying every month that if I'm pregnant, God will help me to be a great mother, and that I will raise my kids to know and love Him.

Maybe it will happen next month . . .

"Could there be something wrong with one of us?" my husband asked. I knew what he was talking about. I'd just found out—yet again—that I wasn't pregnant.

"It's okay, it's only been five months," I said. "A lot of couples try for longer than that." I smiled, trying to reassure him that nothing was wrong.

"I know; but still, it wouldn't hurt to get checked out. Just to make sure . . ." he said. Dan was 32 when we got married, and now he was 36. He didn't want to wait any longer to start a family. He'd been looking forward to being a daddy, and he didn't want to be too old to play ball with his kids.

I said, "Sometimes it takes awhile. I'm sure there's nothing wrong. But if it will make you feel better, go ahead and set an appointment."

So he did. My husband is the type of person who likes to plan things out, and according to his plan, we were supposed to be starting our family now. We'd been married five years and were ready to take on the responsibility of a child. We definitely had the love to give. But so far, no baby was on the way. It's not always easy waiting for God's timetable; but still, I had faith that we would conceive according to God's calendar, not ours.

That week he went to the doctor and had the tests done; everything proved to be okay, which made Dan feel a lot better.

And then, wouldn't you know it, later that same month I made an astonishing discovery. I was pregnant! Finally, we were expecting a baby! All day long I couldn't stop smiling. In my heart I was jumping up and down with joy; but so far, no one knew except God and me. I wanted to take just a little time to let the reality sink in before I shared the good news.

I was amazed by the new life growing inside me. God's timing is divine. By this, I mean that if our baby's conception had occurred earlier, it would not have been the same Micah we have now—it would have been somebody different. Another day, another time would have brought a different set of chromosomes together, creating a person with different looks and a different personality. It's fascinating and mind-boggling when you think about it! And I am so grateful that it all came together on that day. Our Micah is such a blessing.

In the same way, your baby is special to God, even before he or she is conceived. This makes perfect sense, because God isn't bound by time like we are, and He can see straight into the future. He knows all about your baby beforehand—what he'll look like, what he'll like and dislike, and what his special talents will be. More importantly, God has a plan for your baby's life.

A boy named Jeremiah was called by God to be a leader even before his father and mother conceived him. You might wonder, is that a fantasy, or does God really see babies before they are conceived? Look at what God said in Jeremiah 1:5: "I chose you before I formed you in the womb; I set you apart before you were born. I appointed you a prophet to the nations."

History tells us that when Jeremiah grew up, he foretold of God's judgment and the overthrow of Jerusalem, the 70 years of captivity and the promise of restoration of the Jews—fulfilling God's promise that Jeremiah would be a prophet to the nations.

Your Baby's Name Is on God's Calendar

Could your baby have a plan designed by God for his or her life, even before he or she is born? Yes, absolutely. The possibilities are intriguing. Your child may be called to be an evangelist, teacher, music leader, inventor, financier or writer. God sees into the future and He knows what plans He has for your child. Acts 17:24-27 tells us that God made the world and everything in it, that He Himself gives everyone life and breath and has determined our appointed times. Does that strike you like it strikes me? God gives babies life and breath in His appointed time—it's like your baby's birth date is written on God's calendar and He's got the date circled in pink or blue!

Another Scripture that confirms this concept is Ephesians 1:4: "For He chose us in Him, before the foundation of the world." Can you imagine that? You are waiting anxiously for a positive pregnancy test, and God's Word says He has already chosen your child way back before the foundation of the world!

A lovely young woman named Hannah desperately wanted a baby, but it just wasn't happening. After suffering month after month after month of disappointment, she went to the temple to make a plea bargain with God.

"If you will give me a son, I will give him back to you, God," she said.

God was pleased with her faith, and He said, "I'll take you up on that."

God cured the problem that was preventing Hannah from becoming pregnant, and she had a son she named Samuel. True to her promise, she let Samuel grow up in the temple, under the guidance of the prophet Eli; and sure enough, God used Samuel for His purposes. After Eli passed on, Samuel became a great prophet (the first to proclaim the coming of Jesus) and the judge of Israel who restored law and anointed Israel's first king, Saul, and then later replaced him with David, the shepherd boy, according to the instruction of the Lord.

All of this was designed by God, even before Samuel's conception.

If you're still waiting for your pregnancy to happen, now is a good time to pray for God's timing.

Tap Into God's Power for Your Baby

How would you like to have the secret of tapping into God's power? If someone offered to sell you the secret of God's power, wouldn't you do everything you could to come up with the money to buy it? I think most of us would. As simple as it may sound, prayer is the secret for tapping into God's power—and it won't cost you a cent. You see, God said He would work on your behalf when you pray.

It's as if there are wonderful gifts, all wrapped and ready to go, sitting up in heaven waiting for us to take them. All we have to do is pray and receive. But too often we forget about the gifts and don't ask. We worry instead of praying. We talk to our friends, but we don't pray. And it's like God is saying, I'd love to give you some of these fabulous prizes, but you have to ask Me for them, because that's how the spiritual law works.

God works through prayer. And prayer works.

I like to use Scripture in my prayers, because Hebrews 4:12 says the Word of God is "living and effective," which means that when we pray using the Word of God, we're taking part in something that is *alive!* I like that. And it's *effective,* meaning it works. God's power is released when we pray.

Knowing this truth, I prayed to get pregnant, and I prayed for my unborn babies every day of my pregnancies. I prayed for what was going on developmentally each week, and then I asked God for His blessing. As this story unfolds, you'll discover how prayer made all the difference in my pregnancies, my deliveries and in my son and daughter. You can experience God's power for your own life and your baby, too, as you pray.

Here's a promise from God you can hang on to: "Now this is the confidence we have before Him: whenever we ask anything according to His will, He hears us. And if we know that He hears whatever we ask, we know that we have what we have asked Him for" (1 John 5:14-15.) That's a good Scripture to write out and post on your mirror to read every morning before you pray.

How to Pray

Prayer is not complicated, and you don't have to be poetic or use fancy words. Prayer is simply talking to God. You can talk to Him like you talk to your best friend. You can also pray by applying the Scriptures to your situation.

At the end of each chapter is a prayer to start you off. After you read the prayer aloud, continue on, adding your own words. Remember, you don't have to edit and polish up your prayers; just talk to God from your heart. He hears you and He understands. He's got some beautiful gifts waiting for you, so go ahead: ask and receive.

You'll also find Scriptures for thought and meditation and a place for you to journal at the end of each chapter.

A MOTHER'S PRAYER FOR WEEK 1

Dear Lord, I believe You have a divine plan for each of our lives. You know the future and You know the child I am going to have, even now, before I'm pregnant. Jeremiah 1:5 says, "I chose you before I formed you in the womb." I take this as an encouragement that You see into the future and You know the baby I'm going to have. Lord, I pray for Your plan to come to pass and for Your will to be done, even as Your Word says, "I set you apart before you were born."

Lord, let me conceive and be blessed with a healthy pregnancy. Hear my prayer just as You heard the prayer of Hannah. I believe You put that account in the Bible for a reason—so that women such as myself would be encouraged to have faith.

If there is anything preventing me from getting pregnant, I ask for Your healing. You know all things, and You are still doing miracles today. I let go of stress, anxiety and worry; and I will meditate on Your promises instead.

I receive Your peace. Philippians 4:7 says, "the peace of God, which surpasses every thought, will guard your hearts and your minds in Christ Jesus." I thank You for peace.

I choose faith and to trust in You, Lord, for the blessing of pregnancy. I stand on the promise of Your Word. Jesus, You said, "Whatever you ask in My name, I will do it so that the Father may be glorified in the Son. If you ask Me anything in My name, I will do it" (John 14:13-14). I claim that promise for my husband and me, and I ask for a child.

And, Lord, help me be the best mother I can be. Give me the wisdom to raise this child according to Your ways, so that he or she grows to love You and serve You all his or her life.

I thank You now, in advance, for hearing and answering my prayer. I know You have good plans for me and my family. My future and my hope are in You.

In Jesus' name I pray. Amen.

Scriptures for Thought and Meditation

Trust in the Lord with all your heart, and do not rely on your own understanding; think about Him in all your ways, and He will guide you on the right paths.

PROVERBS 3:5-6

Whatever you ask in My name, I will do it so that the Father may be glorified in the Son. If you ask Me anything in My name, I will do it.
JOHN 14:13-14

My Journal

Your writing will serve as a memory you can read with your child later. It's a way you can create a special bond as you look back to the time when you were waiting for him or her to be born.

My thoughts on looking forward to having a baby:

_____
_____
_____
_____
_____
_____
_____
_____
_____
_____
_____
_____
_____
_____
_____
_____
_____
_____
_____
_____
_____
_____
_____
_____

2

Your Body, God's Perfect Vessel

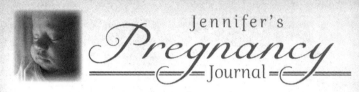

Jennifer's
Pregnancy
Journal

November 22: *It's official. I just got a positive result on the pregnancy test. I can't believe I'm pregnant! I'm so excited! It's Thanksgiving in three days. I'll wait until then and give my husband something to really be thankful for! I can't wait to see the expression on his face. This is going to be the best Thanksgiving ever.*

November 24: *I can't wait till tomorrow. I'm going crazy being the only one who knows I'm pregnant—well, besides God. I've decided how to spring the happy news. I made Dan a card and wrote "To Daddy" on the envelope. Then for the note on the inside, I wrote:*

Dear Daddy, you don't know me yet, but I'm growing inside of Mommy. I can't wait to meet you. I know you're going to be the best father in the world. I know you will love me unconditionally. If I decide to be a garbage collector or a doctor, it will never matter to you. I know you'll always be there for me and always protect me. I love you so much and want to be just like you when I grow up.

Mommy says that you're a very hard worker but that you have a soft side, too. Please be extra nice to Mommy these next nine months, because she's a little scared about what's going to happen with me growing inside of her. Love her and hug her lots, because I can feel it too! I can't wait to meet you, Daddy.
Love, Your Baby

Seventeen years ago, I became a Certified Personal Trainer and nutrition counselor specializing in training for women. Many of my clients have been moms or moms-to-be. I love helping women improve their physical fitness, because it's important to take care of the body God blessed you with. First Corinthians 6:19-20 says, "Do you not know that your body is a sanctuary of the Holy Spirit who is in you, whom you have from God? You are not your own, for you were bought at a price; therefore glorify God in your body."

One of the ways we can glorify God in our body is by respecting it and taking proper care of it. As Christians, we tend to focus mostly on the heart and mind, and forget about the body; so in this short chapter, I want to concentrate on the habitat that will be your baby's home for the next nine months.

Some women who come to me for training aren't real happy with their bodies, and they experience a lot of negative feelings toward themselves as a result. I want to encourage you to put a stop to those derogatory thoughts. Don't look in the mirror and say hateful things about your body. Instead, think about the positive progress you're going to make from here on out, and give yourself the respect that a vessel designed by God deserves. God made your body to be a perfect habitat to nurture, grow and birth your baby; and that is a beautiful miracle.

"But I'm the exception. I wasn't born with a perfect body," someone might say. Please let me share with you a true story about one woman—my own aunt—whose doctor told her as much.

When my aunt, Kimberly Grano, was born, she was premature and weighed just two pounds. Her lungs hadn't had time to fully develop; as a result, she struggled with illness and disabilities throughout her life. Even as an adult, her left lung does not function, and she breathes with only 65 percent of her right lung.

After Kimberly met Gaetano (Guy), the love of her life, and they became engaged, they talked and prayed about how they wanted to have a child together one day. They asked the Lord for His help and for His will to be done. Several months before the wedding, Kimberly visited her OB/GYN for a checkup and told him about her plans for the future.

Both the OB/GYN specialist and her family general practitioner counseled Kimberly and Guy, explaining that because of her medical history, it would take a *very long time* for her to become pregnant—*if it happened ever, at all.*

So the couple continued to pray, and they got married. They didn't know how long it would take, but they believed God for a baby. And guess what happened?

She got pregnant on their honeymoon.

But that's not the end of the story. For the critical first three months, Kimberly bled off and on. The doctor warned her that she could lose the baby.

Kimberly said, "We prayed God's will for our baby's life and for our lives, even more than ever before! We believed God wanted our child to be here and to be a part of His divine purpose and plan."

After nine months, Kimberly gave birth to a beautiful baby girl, born full-term and healthy. She wrote, "Thank You, heavenly Father, Jesus, and Holy Spirit for Your wonderful and amazing gifts of love and life! And for answered prayer!"

Even though my aunt was born with physical problems herself, she *was* God's perfect vessel for her baby girl, my cousin Gina.

God's Help Is Available to You

When you're pregnant or soon-to-be pregnant, it's important to treat your body with care and respect, because you are bringing a new life into the world, and this little person is totally dependent on you for his or her health. This is an awesome responsibility. I encourage you to take it seriously and to ask God for His help.

Even if you have a history of bad habits, such as eating unhealthy foods and ignoring exercise, you can turn that around now by making a commitment and claiming God's promise in Philippians 4:13: "I am able to do all things through Him who strengthens me." At the end of this chapter is a prayer to help you do this.

This reminds me of a client I had who was already a mother of two children, and now she was expecting again. She told me she had a difficult time her first two pregnancies, and she wanted it to be different this time. Under my guidance, she ate healthy, worked out and prayed; and you know what happened? She said her third pregnancy was the easiest and best pregnancy experience—by far! She could hardly believe how much easier her delivery was and how quickly she bounced back afterward, because she took good care of herself. So no matter where you are right now in your physical and spiritual health, this is the perfect time for you to soar ahead to new heights—using good principles of health, prayer and reliance on God's strength. Here are five important tips I shared with her that will help you during your pregnancy too.

Five Vital Tips for Taking Care of Your Body, God's Vessel

1. Support Your Pregnancy with Proper Nutrition

Expectant moms need about 300 more calories a day for a single birth and 600 calories for twins.[1] Don't fall into the trap of thinking, *I'm going to gain weight anyway, so this is my chance to eat whatever I feel like eating.* Everything you put into your body goes to your baby too. I believe eating unhealthy food is a form of abusing your unborn child, just like smoking or drinking alcohol is a form of abusing your baby.

Here is a quick overview. Protein is critical for growth and necessary for your baby's brain cells. Pregnant women need 75 to 100 grams of protein a day. Fruits and vegetables high in vitamin C help ensure your baby's bone and tooth development and help manufacture collagen, which holds tissue together and helps in an easier delivery. Carbohydrates provide necessary fuel for your body and your baby's body, and have been known to help with morning sickness.

2. Take Folate and Prenatal Vitamins *Now*

Folate, or folic acid, is a B vitamin that's necessary to help prevent neural tube defects like spina bifida during the first trimester. Women who plan to get pregnant need to start taking it immediately, because your baby needs it from day one. The U.S. Public Health Service recommends 400 micrograms a day.

Take a good prenatal vitamin to ensure your baby gets all the key nutrients. If one brand makes you feel nauseated, switching to another, more gentle formula may help.

3. Form the Water Habit

Our bodies are more than two-thirds water, and our brains are more than 80 percent water. Your unborn baby is surrounded by water, and your body needs water to produce a healthy baby. I recommend drinking at least eight 8-ounce glasses of water a day. Guard against becoming dehydrated, as that's one of the worst things you could do for you and your baby.

4. Exercise as You Are Able

Exercise is magnificent for relieving stress and helping cope with wild mood swings caused by pregnancy hormones. When you exercise consistently, you'll gain a sense of empowerment and being in control of your body and your life. You might walk with a friend or use the time to talk with God about your baby.

Make sure you follow your physician's recommendation for exercise. Every woman and pregnancy is unique, so exercise only according to what is healthy and safe for you.

5. Indulge in Rest and Sleep

Don't feel bad about craving sleep. It's perfectly normal, because your body is going through so many changes, especially in the first trimester. Toward the end of your pregnancy, it gets harder to find a comfortable way to sleep, and I can't help but believe that God is getting a new mother ready for the nights of interrupted sleep she'll have after her baby arrives.

There isn't enough space in one short chapter to provide complete information about nutrition and exercise during pregnancy. For more details, please see my website, www.Pray ForYourBaby.com.

My prayer for you this week is that you'll find new joy in taking good care of your body and peace in knowing that you are respecting the perfect vessel God gave you.

A Mother's Prayer for Week 2

Dear Lord,

Help me respect the body You gave me. I make a commitment today to treat it right by following principles of good nutrition and by exercising. Help me keep this commitment, even when it's hard and I don't feel like it. Your Word says the body is the sanctuary of the Holy Spirit; so, God, help me treat my body with the care it deserves. When I'm tempted to eat unhealthy junk food, help me be strong and resist temptation. When I'm tempted to be lazy and skip exercise, help me take hold of Scriptures, like "I am able to do all things through Him who strengthens me" (Philippians 4:13). Be my strength and my motivation, God.

I will not give in to bulimia or starvation diets, which can be harmful or fatal to my unborn baby. I will look to You for a healthy self-image, Lord. I will not give in to binge eating and overeating. I will look to You for a healthy lifestyle, Lord. John 8:32 says, "You will know the truth, and the truth will set you free." I claim this promise for my own, and that I will be free of all ungodly, unhealthy eating habits.

I will value my body and treat it right. I will meditate on Your Word for strength.

Psalm 27:11 says, "Teach me your way, O LORD" (NIV). I pray that You would teach me how to live, day by day, according to Your ways, using Your strength.

I pray for good health for myself and for my baby, and to reflect a good Christian witness in all I do.

In Jesus' name. Amen.

Scriptures for Thought and Meditation

My help comes from the LORD, the Maker of heaven and earth.
PSALM 121:2

I am able to do all things through Him who strengthens me.
PHILIPPIANS 4:13

My Journal

How I am taking good care of my body as God's vessel:

_____

_____

_____

_____

_____

_____

_____

_____

What I can do to establish a healthy diet and exercise regimen:

_____

_____

_____

_____

_____

_____

What I want my child to learn from me about healthy living:

_____

_____

_____

_____

_____

_____

_____

_____

Note

1. The American College of Obstetrics and Gynecology. http://www.acog.org/publications/patient_education/bp103.cfm.

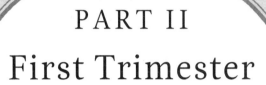

PART II

First Trimester

(WEEKS 3 TO 12)

*This is the word of the L*ORD *your Maker
who shaped you from birth;
He will help you.*
ISAIAH 44:2

3

It's a Miracle!

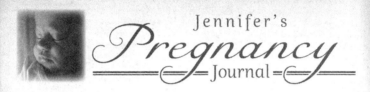

Jennifer's
Pregnancy
Journal

Wednesday, the day before Thanksgiving: My homemade card with the baby announcement inside is all ready to give to Dan. I'm so excited to give it to him that I just can't wait any longer! I know he won't be expecting this right now, and I can't wait to see his face when he reads the card. I just have to tell him. Okay, I've made a decision . . . I'm giving him the card TONIGHT!

We'd both had a hard day. Dan called me from work earlier and said he'd just lost another client. The timing couldn't have been worse. The holidays were coming up, and money was already tight. In fact, we didn't know how we were going to pay all the bills—let alone have the finances for a new baby. When Dan came home from work, I tried to act like everything was okay.

"How was your day, babe?" I asked.

"Not great. I'm just glad we have this four-day weekend to enjoy with some good food!" he said.

"Me too."

I placed the card on Dan's dinner plate as he went downstairs to his office to check his email. I finished getting dinner ready and then called down to him, "Come and eat. Dinner's ready."

He came upstairs and sat down at his usual place at the table. He looked at the card in front of him that had the words "To Daddy" written on the envelope. I held my breath, waiting for his reaction. I saw tears come to his eyes.

"Are we—? I mean, how—?" He was trying to wrap his head around what he read on the envelope as he opened it up. I couldn't stand the suspense any longer.

"YES!" I said, now crying too.

"But how, how, how can we be pregnant?" Dan said. We both knew that this month we had only "tried" one time, and even then it wasn't anywhere near the prime date to conceive; so this was truly a surprise.

"It's a miracle!" I said. I believe it was truly God's way of telling us that He is in control—like He always is.

As soon as Dan got to the last line of my special note, he launched out of his chair and dashed around the table to give me the biggest hug. And then there we were in each other's arms, laughing and praising God, with tears of joy running down our cheeks.

"I'm so happy," he said, over and over again. I'll never forget that moment, announcing the news of our coming baby to my husband. He was beyond thrilled, and by the time we sat down in our chairs again, we both had tears of joy in our eyes.

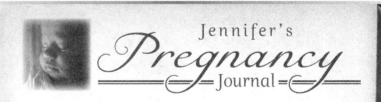

Jennifer's

Pregnancy

Journal

November 25: It's a boy! Don't ask me how I know, but I do. I just have this feeling that God is blessing us with a baby boy. I told Dan, and from the look on his face, I don't think he totally believes me, but he'll find out soon enough! I know I'm right.

Something of major importance happens in that very first second when you become pregnant. The sex of your baby is chosen. Can you imagine what that means? At that very moment, even before there is a head and body or a recognizable shape, there is a male or female in the making.

One cell of life, just one second old . . . and yet so much is already determined.

After I told my husband we were expecting, I looked at him and smiled.

"It's a boy," I said, as if I'd been safeguarding a wonderful secret and was now letting him in on the news. Dan wasn't so sure. We agreed not to find out the sex of our baby until the birth, so we had lots of time to wait and wonder.

You may or may not have a feeling about your baby being a boy or girl; nonetheless, it's already determined from that first moment of conception. Biology tells us that the mother's egg has an X sex chromosome, and the father's sperm can have either an X or a Y sex chromosome. If the father's X meets up with the mother's egg, you'll have a girl. If his Y chromosome meets up with the mother's egg, you'll have a boy. Whether you believe the selection of chromosomes that determines the sex of your baby is random or specifically determined by God, no one can dispute the fact that it is the father's chromosome that determines whether your baby is a boy or a girl.

Within hours of conception, that single cell formed by your X and the daddy's Y or X has divided again and again. Just a few days later, this microscopic bundle of cells, which is about one-fifth the size of the dot over this letter *i*, is cruising through your fallopian tube to the warm, nourishing space that will be his or her internal nursery—your uterus. Once there, it takes about six days for your newly conceived baby to settle in and start getting nourishment from you through your bloodstream. Everything you eat—from that nutritious green salad to those fat-soaked, salt-drenched fries—is going into the tiny baby that is doing its best to grow and be healthy. Something else is happening too.

Your baby takes in the nutrition and releases the human gonadotropin hormone (HCG) into your bloodstream. This can cause all kinds of surprises—you're suddenly zapped of energy and want to take naps, or you can no longer stand certain smells, or your stomach turns inside out, or you feel hyperemotional and get into an argument with someone you love over the tiniest, most unimportant thing.

And then it dawns on you. *Could it be? Could I be pregnant?*

If you haven't already begun, now is the time to start praying for your pregnancy and your baby. Even today, when I think back to how the Holy Spirit led me to pray for Micah while he was still growing inside me, I can't help but get tears in my eyes, because I am seeing the results of those nine months of prayer every day in my son. And I can say the same thing for my second baby, my daughter, Malia Grace. God has granted many of the specific things I prayed for. For example, you'll read later how I asked God to help my son memorize Scripture and how, at 24 months, Micah could recite the entire twenty-third psalm.

Prayer is ordained by God, and we are instructed in the holy Bible to pray. Even Jesus, God's Son, the Anointed One prayed. Be encouraged about prayer for you and your baby, because prayer has worked for me and for so many others; you'll read their stories here.

Dutch Sheets is a respected theologian and author of *Intercessory Prayer,* a book that reveals "how God can use your prayers to move heaven and earth." Pastor Sheets wrote, "God works through the prayers of His people. . . . Without question, humans were forever to be God's link to authority and activity on the earth. Here we have, I believe, the reason for the necessity of prayer. God chose, from the time of the Creation, to work on the earth through humans, not independent of them. He always has and always will, even at the cost of becoming one. Though God is sovereign and all-powerful, Scripture clearly tells us that he limited Himself, concerning the affairs of Earth, to working *through* human beings."[1]

This is why I feel compelled to share the importance of prayer with you. I believe that God wants mothers today, more than ever, to begin praying for their sons and daughters right from the very start—before they are born. As the parent of your child, God has given you the authority to claim the biblical promises on his or her behalf. You have the power to give your baby the advantage of prayer starting right now.

Give Your Baby a Head Start Through Prayer

It's popular to give children a head start in learning, and parents often teach their children at home before they're old enough to go to school. Moms enroll their children in special classes for music and foreign language and many other areas of knowledge. But what about giving your child a head start even before he or she is born, through the awesome power of prayer—prayer that is Bible-based and faith-driven and led by the Holy Spirit? When you realize the power of praying for your unborn child, believe me, you won't want to hold back.

A MOTHER'S PRAYER FOR WEEK 3

Dear Heavenly Father,

Thank You for the child You are giving me. Thank You for this awesome miracle of new life. You are the only one who knows if I am having a boy or a girl, and whichever it is, I ask for You to bless my baby with good health and with love.

Lord, please help me feel well physically, and take away any morning sickness or other hardships that may make it hard for me to concentrate on You and this gift You are giving me.

I pray against miscarriage, Jesus. I know how common it is, but I know You want me to have a healthy baby, and so I claim a healthy pregnancy, in Jesus' name.

I know love is the most important gift I can give my baby, so help me to be the most loving mother I can be. Father God, I want to be an extension of Your love. Use me to bring Your love into my child's life. Anoint me to teach my child how to pray. Help me teach my child Your ways and Your Word. Help me be a good role model. And again, I praise You for this wonderful miracle of life that's growing inside me.

In Jesus' name I pray. Amen.

Scriptures for Thought and Meditation

Acknowledge that the LORD is God. He made us, and we are His.
PSALM 100:3

*Lord, You have searched me and known me. You know when I sit down
and when I stand up: You understand my thoughts from far away. You
observe my travels and my rest; You are aware of all my ways.*
PSALM 139:1-3

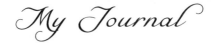

I discovered I was pregnant when:

_____

_____

_____

_____

_____

_____

_____

_____

_____

_____

How I told my husband:

_____

_____

_____

_____

_____

_____

_____
_____
_____
_____

I think I'm having a boy/girl because:

_____
_____
_____
_____
_____
_____
_____
_____
_____
_____

I want to know/be surprised about the gender of my baby because:

_____
_____
_____
_____
_____
_____
_____
_____
_____
_____

Note
1. Dutch Sheets, *Intercessory Prayer: How God Can Use Your Prayers to Move Heaven and Earth* (Ventura, CA: Regal, 1996), pp. 28-29.

4

The Beginning of Your Baby's Brain

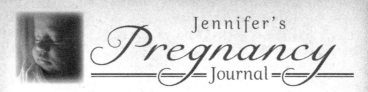

We just found out we're pregnant for the second time, and I couldn't wait to tell someone. I made plans to meet my girl-friend who now lives in Florida but is back for a visit. I haven't seen her in a while, and I thought this would be a good chance to catch up.

We met for lunch, and I told her about a book idea that came to me in the middle of the night. I said, "I believe God wants me to write a book to inspire and encourage women to pray for their unborn babies."

"I love that idea!" she replied. "You know, I prayed for each of my three children when I was pregnant, and I can see my prayers still being answered, even today, 15 years later."

We had such fun chatting over lunch. We hugged and said good-bye. My head was swirling with thoughts and ideas about the book, and I was so excited about being pregnant that I wanted to announce to everyone I passed, "I'm pregnant!" I was so distracted from what I was doing, which was getting two-year-old Micah strapped in to his car seat and ready to go, that I fastened his seat belt, tossed the car keys onto the front seat and shut the door. Just then, I had a very bad feeling.

Sure enough, I lifted my door handle and discovered the door was locked! Oh my goodness, poor little Micah was locked inside the car with the keys on the front seat where he couldn't reach them. He couldn't unbuckle himself, and it was almost 100 degrees on that July day.

I sprinted into the restaurant, crying, and found the hostess. "I just locked my son in the hot car! And I'm pregnant! I need help, quick!"

Immediately, I called 911, and EVERYONE came rushing to the scene in about three minutes flat. There was the pumper truck that always goes to car accidents, the giant hook-and-ladder truck, AND the ambulance. I was so embarrassed! But, thank God, they arrived quickly, so I didn't have to break a window. Dan would have died. But there was Micah, smiling at the firemen the whole time they worked on the doors. It actually took awhile to get in, but Micah was just fine—just a little thirsty, but so excited to be saved by the nice firemen.

What a day! My brain is NOT working right!!!

Your baby is just 14 days old, and yet something of monumental importance is happening. A sheet of cells is rapidly growing into what will become your baby's brain, spinal cord and backbone. Why these three? The answer is fascinating.

The brain is going to control everything your child does—from involuntary breathing, to talking, to balancing on a bicycle and learning to read. Although the brain gives instructions to the body, it can't do its job alone; it needs a long bundle of nerves to relay messages to (and from) the various parts of the body. These tireless "message senders" are located inside the spinal column, which is protected by the vertebrae. It's a complex and beautiful design engineered by our Creator God.

As if this isn't enough going on, the placenta and umbilical cord have already been forming as well.[1] So don't be surprised if you feel like sleeping more than usual. I know I did. When I was pregnant with Micah, I was still working as a personal trainer, and sometimes I'd sneak into the back room or my car and take a mini-nap between appointments with clients. Other days, I'd get home from work and collapse on the couch, which is totally not like me, because I'm a high-energy person who likes to get up and go. I never nap during the day unless I'm sick. And during those first few weeks, I'd sleep in, and at times, I never even got out of my PJs. Thank goodness that didn't last too long.

You might find yourself out of your normal routine, and that's okay; because once your new baby comes, your routine is going to be interrupted a lot! So for me, I just figured this was God's way of preparing me to be flexible. On the other hand, some women don't feel sick or tired or any different at all during their first weeks of pregnancy; and if that's the case for you, don't worry—consider yourself blessed. Every pregnancy is unique, just as God made each of us unique.

The one thing we can all do as moms and moms-to-be is to pray for our babies now. Jesus said, "If you ask Me anything in My name, I will do it" (John 14:14). Isn't that a fantastic promise? That's why I like to end my prayers with the phrase "in Jesus' name, amen." It's like saying, "By the authority of Jesus I pray, so be it."

I also suggest that you have a regular time of day for praying, because when prayer becomes part of your routine, you don't forget. Some people like to say a short prayer as soon as they wake up, even before they get out of bed. You might look at the clock and say, "Thank You, Lord, for this day. I believe You're going to help me make it a wonderful day. Lead me and guide me, and bless my baby." And so on. Then you get up knowing the Holy Spirit is right with you. There's no "getting up on the wrong side of the bed" when you start your day with Jesus!

Or, you might be one of those people who need time to wake up, and midday or evening prayer works better. I know one young woman who goes for a walk every day on a path through the woods near her home and spends that time out in nature talking to God. So in addition to a formal prayer, you can also talk to God throughout your day while you're folding the towels or whatever. Make Him your confidant and best friend.

I like to pray aloud. Maybe you will want to do that too, because as you'll read later, your baby is able to hear your voice before he or she is born. I met a lady at my hair salon recently, and we started talking about how important it is to pray for your baby. She told me that during her pregnancy, she read the *entire* Bible to her baby. Her daughter is now 16 years old, and she has a remarkable love and desire for the Word of God. I just love that! What a wonderful way to give your child the Bible even before he or she is born!

Along with the fact that at some point in the pregnancy your baby can hear your voice, I believe that your baby also bonds with you even before he or she is born by becoming accustomed to your voice. Although your baby can't hear you yet, it's good to get in the habit of audible prayer. I also like to pray out loud because hearing the prayers that incorporate the power of God's Word bolsters my faith. So even though God can hear your thoughts, I recommend praying aloud sometimes too. When you speak aloud God's truth through prayer, you release the power of God to work in your life. And as you hear yourself speak, your faith is strengthened as well.

When you grasp the realization that you can tap into a divine resource through prayer, you understand the power you have at your disposal. God wants you to use this power to bring His will to pass in your life; so this week, pray for God to bless your baby's progress as the brain, spinal cord and backbone are forming. And since we're on the topic of prayer, pray that your baby will grow up to be a man or woman of prayer.

Both my coauthor, Carolyn, and I were taught to pray by our mothers. Prayer is a wonderful legacy we all can pass on to our children—the faith and knowledge that God works through prayer.

A Mother's Prayer for Week 4

Dear Lord, thank You for this baby that's growing inside me. I can't quite understand what is going on with my baby at this moment, so I give it to You and ask You to bless it. Lord, please help my baby's brain develop perfectly, and give my baby wisdom beyond his years.

God, You are the Creator of all life. I pray now that this baby will grow normally, just as it is supposed to, according to Your plan for pregnancy. I pray that the cells will multiply and grow and that the brain and spinal cord will develop properly. Give my baby a strong spinal cord and a strong, intelligent mind.

Jesus, You said to ask for what we need, in Your name, and You would do it. You said it and I believe it. Therefore, I am obeying Your Word by asking You to bless my baby's growth and make my baby healthy and strong.

And, Lord, I pray that my son or daughter will grow up to be a person of prayer—that he or she will have faith and tap into Your power through prayer.

I pray in the name of the Father God, Jesus Christ and the Holy Spirit. Amen.

Scriptures for Thought and Meditation

Every generous act and every perfect gift is from above, coming down from the Father of lights.
JAMES 1:17

I assure you: Anything you ask the Father in My name, He will give you. Until now you have asked for nothing in My name. Ask and you will receive, that your joy may be complete.
JOHN 16:23-24

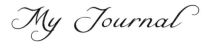

The best time of the day (or night), and the best place for me to consistently pray for my baby:

_____

_____

_____

_____

_____

_____

_____

_____

_____

_____

Matthew 21:22 encourages me because:

_____

_____

_____

_____

_____

_____

_____

_____

My thoughts about God using me to create a new life:

_____

_____

_____

_____

_____

_____

_____

_____

_____

Note

1. "The Development of a Foetus," Natracare. http://www.natracare.com/help_for_schools/ fact_files/ks4/reproduction_the_development_of_a_foetus_ks4.htm.

5

God Hears Your Baby's Heartbeat

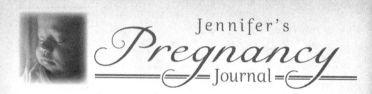

Jennifer's *Pregnancy* Journal

It just hit me: I'm both happy and scared at the realization that I'm going to be a mommy. We called our family and told them the big news, and they are all excited for us. My dad is probably the most excited, and that means so much to me. Dad and I have had our differences over the years, so this is really special to have him on my side.

It was so much fun announcing to our friends and clients that we are going to have a baby. Everyone is excited for us, and they say they can't wait to see the baby with muscles (because Dan and I are both trainers and fitness coaches).

One thing I'm looking forward to is hearing the baby's heartbeat. I know that will be special for Dan too.

By five weeks, your baby's heart has started beating. Your doctor probably won't hear it with a stethoscope yet, but ultrasound machines have detected movement of a baby's heart at this point in the pregnancy. Just think: God hears your baby's heart beating! Remember, God said He knows us before we're born, and He is very much aware of the baby growing rapidly inside you.

By next week, it will beat about 150 times a minute and remain at that heart rate until birth. After your baby is born, the heart pumps blood to every cell in the body in less than 60 seconds, every second for a lifetime. Just how many heartbeats does that add up to? One estimate, based on averages, is 2.8 billion heartbeats—now that's what I call an example of God's creative power![1]

A Baby with No Heartbeat

My friend Darla Sanborn was thrilled when she found out she was expecting her second baby. Against all medical odds, God had blessed the Sanborns with a son, and they desperately wanted another child; so when she and her husband learned that Darla was pregnant again, they were overjoyed. Then the unthinkable happened.

At her six-week checkup and ultrasound, the physician said, "I'm sorry, Mrs. Sanborn, but you've lost the baby. You will miscarry soon." Darla didn't want to accept that verdict. She felt certain that she was pregnant with a live baby, so she requested a second ultrasound.

Her doctor performed another ultrasound, taking extra care to locate a beating heart, but the verdict remained the same—the baby had no heartbeat and her pregnancy could not continue. Darla was sent home to wait for her body to miscarry her baby.

But Darla didn't do that; instead, she went home and prayed and expected her baby to live. She also asked her church to join in prayer. Then Darla packed up her toddler and went to visit her mother in Tennessee, for more support. Her mother and her mother's church also joined in prayer and faith, believing God to turn this verdict around. In addition, Darla asked friends to pray, and those friends passed on the prayer request to their churches. So, she had entire communities of Christians from Colorado to Tennessee standing in faith for her, proclaiming God's promises in Scripture—praying for her unborn baby.

There is power in receiving the prayer support of others. Jesus said, "Again, I assure you: If two of you on earth agree about any matter that you pray for, it will be done for you by My Father in heaven. For where two or three are gathered together in My name, I am there among them" (Matthew 18:19-20). Darla had many more than two or three praying—so would this make a difference?

Darla and her mother had faith that it would.

After two weeks had passed and she still hadn't miscarried, her mother said, "Let's take you to see an OB/GYN here in town."

So another ultrasound was performed; there it was right on the monitor—the baby's heart, beating just as it should. Her baby was alive!

Now there's more to Darla's story coming up in the next chapter, but first, let's take a look at what else is happening with your baby's development this week.

A Heart of Love

One of the personal things Darla shared with me is that her son portrays a genuine heart of love, and people who meet him often remark on what a kind, loving person he is. His love for life and his love for others shine through his eyes.

This week, while you're praying for your baby's physical heart, I also want you to pray that he or she will grow up with a heart of love for God and others. Jesus said, "I have spoken these things to you so that My joy may be in you and your joy may be complete. This is My command: love one another as I have loved you" (John 15:11-12).

Jesus repeated this command several times, showing us how important it is to have a heart of love for others. So we learn that loving others with a Christlike love is one way to bring joy into our life.

A MOTHER'S PRAYER FOR WEEK 5

Dear Father God, thank You for this wonderful miracle of life You have given me. May joy and gladness fill my heart and spill over to everyone who hears the good news of my pregnancy. A new baby is a blessing for the whole family, so I pray that our parents will be blessed by the news of having this grandbaby. I pray that the uncles and aunties will be blessed and filled with joy. And for all our friends and loved ones, let them share in our joy and gratitude. I pray that this time of rejoicing and gladness would also be a time of praising You for Your blessing of the miracle of life. Your Word says that every good and perfect gift comes from above, so I give You my thanks for this wonderful gift.

I thank You for my baby's heartbeat, and even though I can't hear it yet, I know You can. Bless my baby's heart and cause it to grow strong, just as it should be. Protect my baby's heart from any defects or problems. Your Word says that in the beginning, Your creative powers were at work. I acknowledge Your power and ask You to extend it to my baby also. Create a healthy baby, week by week, as he (or she) grows.

And, Lord, give my child a heart to love and serve You. Give my child a tender heart, open to hearing Your voice, and to be kind and compassionate toward others. Please help me to be a good role model of these attitudes as well. Help me lead my child in prayer and in opening up our hearts to You to receive Your love.

In Jesus' name I pray. Amen.

Scriptures for Thought and Meditation

Man does not see what the LORD sees, for man sees what is visible, but the Lord sees the heart.
1 SAMUEL 16:7

God, create a clean heart for me and renew a steadfast spirit within me.
PSALM 51:10

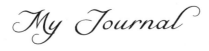

My Journal

The first people I announced my pregnancy to:

_____

_____

_____

_____

_____

_____

_____

_____

How they responded to the news:

_____

_____

_____

_____

_____

_____

The ways I chose to share the news of my pregnancy (Twitter, Facebook or phone calls; or traditional communication, such as letters or email; or my thoughts on why I kept my pregnancy private):

_____

_____

_____

_____

_____

_____

_____

_____

Note

1. A heart beats about 70 times/minute. An average life span is about 75 years. 75 years x (70 heartbeats/minute) = 75 years x (36,792,000 beats/year). That equals about 2,800,000,000 beats. Malcolm Swan, Mathematics Education, University of Nottingham and Jim Ridgway, School of Education, "Tools-Math Plausible Estimation Estimating Facts Tasks, Set#2," http://www.flaguide.org/tools/math/estimation/amazing facts1B.php.

6

Your Baby's Face

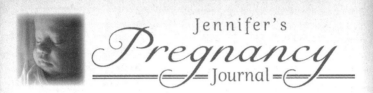

Jennifer's
Pregnancy
Journal

I started my video journal this week to record all the details of my pregnancy. I am getting more excited about having a baby! I wonder what he/she will look like. I bet he'll have dark hair like his father. And what color eyes? Probably brown, like both of ours. Will he have a dimple like me? I can't wait to see my baby's face! I know that both Dan and I are going to go crazy with the camera once our little one makes his appearance, especially me—I love photography.

It's December now, and we'll be going to visit Dan's sister in California for Christmas this year. We always have a great time, but I wish we were also going to see my family in Hawaii. I really want to be with my mom during this special time in my life. I have a lot of questions, and if anyone can answer them it's her—she's had seven kids!

By the end of this week, you will officially have been pregnant for one month—and your baby has grown to triple its size. He or she is now about 1/8 inch long. Still tiny, but so much is going on; and what I think is exciting is that your baby's facial features are beginning to take shape.

Your baby is taking after you or your husband, or a little of both, all according to the directions spelled out in the unique combination of genes you've both provided. Here's what's going on:

• The beginning of eyes and ears develop with the openings in just the right places.

• A tiny space for the mouth appears.
• Your baby's stomach and lungs are beginning to form.
• Small buds that will grow into arms and legs take shape.

Talk about a growth spurt! Don't feel bad if you're still craving sleep.

This week, we want to pray for the magnificent growth that is taking place in your baby and, specifically, for the development of self-respect that will be manifested in the facial expression your child portrays to the world—a first impression he or she will project throughout life. When children are young, you can see how they're feeling just by looking at their faces. A toddler doesn't hide a pout or a feeling of sheer delight. It's only as we get older that we learn to mask our feelings.

When you meet someone, one of the first things you intuit and judge that person by is his or her face. Your idea of that person's personality and sense of self often happens in a millisecond impression of the person's facial expression. Think of someone whose face presents a strong sense of self-respect. I'm sure you can think of people who have a face that portrays self-confidence regardless of "beauty" or lack of it. Perhaps such an image that comes to mind is your grandma. She may be 80 years old, with a vast web of lines and creases on her face, and yet, she portrays self-respect that manifests to the world an attractive self-confidence.

I prayed for my children to grow up with self-respect, and I am doing my best to teach them this concept as they go through different stages of growth. So self-respect is the characteristic I want you to pray for your baby this week, along with his or her physical development.

Now here is the rest of Darla's faith-inspiring story of answered prayer—as I promised in the last chapter.

Darla's Miracle Babies

According to medical science, Darla is not able to have children for three reasons. First, her body does not ovulate, which is necessary for conception. Second, her body does not produce progesterone, the hormone necessary to sustain a pregnancy. And third, she has a subseptate uterus, meaning it's divided in two and would make carrying a baby full-term more challenging—if she were able to get pregnant in the first place. This was devastating news to a woman who had always dreamed of having a family.

And so she began infertility treatment. Her doctor warned her that even with treatment she only had a chance of 1 in 10,000 of getting pregnant. Time went by without a successful pregnancy, and Darla was ready to give up and take a break from the emotional stress.

Family, friends and church members prayed and continued to pray for Darla.

Then, against all odds, on New Year's Day, she conceived. It was a one-time ovulation, and it occurred just when her husband was home from business travel. Nine months later, she gave birth to a baby boy—something her doctor said her body was not able to do.

When God decides to answer a prayer, it doesn't matter how bad the odds are stacked against you. Jesus said to His followers, "With men this is impossible, but with God all things are possible" (Matthew 19:26).

Today, both of Darla's sons are healthy boys and are enrolled in a school program for gifted children. Darla tells them, "God has a purpose for you being here."

I know God has a purpose for your baby, too, just as He has for each and every person.

Let's pray for everything that's happening with your baby's development this week, especially for the reflection of inner strength—honor and self-respect—that will be manifested on your baby's face for all the world to see. We know God answers prayer.

A Mother's Prayer for Week 6

Dear Lord, I am so amazed at the miracle of life that's growing inside me. So much is happening for my baby this week. I just ask that

You watch over him or her and cause the development to go just the way it should. Lord, I pray for my baby's face—the eyes, ears, nose and mouth. Let the face grow perfectly, just the way it's supposed to. And form those features in a way that will reveal inner strength and outer love. And I pray for the internal parts—the stomach and lungs, and the heart and brain. Let them develop into strong, healthy parts for my baby. And last, I pray for the arms and legs to grow just right. Bless my baby in every way: physically, mentally and spiritually. Give my baby a pure, kind heart and a good soul, open to Your Holy Spirit, and to loving You.

I pray that my child will have a healthy sense of self-respect and honor. Help me to teach my child these values and be a good role model of respect and honor. Lord, as a family, we want to portray a Christlike spirit and earn the respect of our community and be a good representative for You.

Once again, I thank You for this wonderful miracle.

I pray in Jesus' name. Amen.

Scriptures for Thought and Meditation

With God all things are possible.
MATTHEW 19:26

Call to Me and I will answer you and tell you great and wondrous things you do not know.
JEREMIAH 33:3

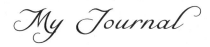

My Journal

My prediction for my baby's hair color and eyes, and my prayer of what will be my baby's first impression on others:

_____

_____

_____

_____

_____

_____

_____

_____

_____

_____

_____

I hope my baby inherits these features and qualities from me and from his/her father:

_____

_____

_____

_____

_____

_____

_____

_____

_____

The person who I most respect and honor, and my reasons for why I respect and honor that person, are as follows:

_____

_____

_____

_____

_____

_____

_____

_____

_____

7

Kidneys, Your Baby's Filtering System

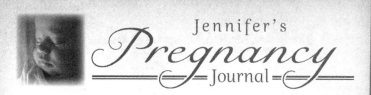

Jennifer's *Pregnancy* Journal

I'm so-o-o-o-o-o tired this week. I feel as if I've been run over by a bus. It's weird because I usually have a lot of energy and am the kind of person who keeps on going all day long!!! But all I want to do is crawl up in a little ball and sleep.

Dan came home the other day and saw me on the couch in the middle of the day when I had a break. He's like, "What's wrong with you?"

I tried to explain how I felt, but I know he didn't get it. I've never experienced anything like this before. I hope I get some energy soon . . .

Please, God, help me get some energy soon. In Psalm 46:10, Your Word says to "be still and know that I am God." I trust that You will help me get through this season of pregnancy. My strength is in You, Lord.

Don't be surprised if you want a nap more than you want to go shopping. This week, your baby is 10,000 times larger than it was at conception—and your body is making that happen.

Not only is your baby growing at hyper-speed, but he or she is also generating new brain cells at the mind-boggling rate of 100 cells per minute. By the time your baby is born, he or she will have about 100 billion neurons, which are the nerve cells that speed messages to and from the brain at the rate of up to 200 miles per hour.

Something else has been happening. Your baby has developed and gone through three sets of kidneys already; and now he has his final set of kidneys—the ones that will remain with him for life. I've never heard anyone give or receive a compliment on the kidneys, but we have to appreciate the service they provide.

The kidneys are sophisticated reprocessing machines designed by God for the important task of filtering out the garbage; and they are at work, even now, while your baby is still developing. In addition, kidneys release three hormones that do the following:

- Stimulate bone marrow to make red blood cells
- Regulate blood pressure
- Help maintain calcium for bones and normal chemical balance in the body

Even though your baby has kidneys, they won't be visible for several more weeks. If you have an ultrasound at week 16 or thereafter, one of the things on the list of items to be examined will be the kidneys.

When I was praying about this chapter and doing basic research on this set of vital organs, it occurred to me that in order to be healthy, we need a spiritual garbage filter as well. I want my son and daughter to filter out the garbage in this world: the ungodly movies, blasphemous internet content, and any other vehicles that carry wrong concepts and ideas to their minds, and lies of all kinds.

Before I gave my life to Jesus Christ, I didn't always stay away from the sins of the world; but, thank God, I came around. I prayed for God to forgive and heal me of my past sins, and that I would not carry on bad habits to my son or daughter. We have all sinned and come short of the glory of God; but when we confess our sins, He wipes them away, and it's like having a clean slate (see Romans 3:23; 1 John 1:9). It's fantastic to know that we can claim victory over every area of temptation, in the name of Jesus. If you've never experienced God's forgiveness, and you're feeling God's urge to know more about it, feel free to skip ahead and read the last chapter now.

Today let's pray for your children to be wise as serpents and harmless as doves (see Matthew 10:16), to be knowing and yet innocent of evil. There's power in praying protection over your unborn baby.

Here's another true account of God answering prayer, which was sent to me by Karen Johnson, a woman who was faithful to pray for her daughter's pregnancy.

Karen's Story

During my daughter Haley's pregnancy, we had several scares.

Early on, the doctor informed her she was a carrier for cystic fibrosis, a heartbreaking disease that shortens the life expectancy of the child. If Haley's husband was also a carrier, there would be a one in four chance the baby would have it. We prayed and we waited the two long weeks to get the results of her husband's blood work—and, praise God, it came back negative.

Then when Haley was six months pregnant, she was set to fly from Chicago to Denver for her brother's wedding. The day before, she received a call from her doctor's office telling her to head straight to the office of a specialist. Evidently there was a problem with one of her tests. Haley called me in tears, not knowing what the problem was. Immediately, I went down on my knees in prayer.

It turned out she had placenta previa, an uncommon condition where the placenta is lying unusually low or blocking the cervix. If this persists, it can cause severe bleeding, require early delivery, and lead to other complications. The doctor watched her closely, and we prayed and waited. God heard us, and her placenta moved in the place it should have been.

As if that wasn't enough drama, a later test revealed a marker for Down's syndrome. Haley and her husband saw no reason to investigate this matter further, as they would not terminate the pregnancy for any reason, so we all continued to pray and trust in God. After the last two scares, I must say that I felt God's peace about whatever was to come. It was like when Jesus said, "Peace I leave with you. My peace I give to you. I do not give to you as the world gives. Your heart must not be troubled or fearful" (John 14:27).

Finally, the day came for Haley to give birth. I thank God that I was able to watch the delivery of my beautiful, perfectly formed granddaughter in February 2005. God is so good! He answers prayers.

A Mother's Prayer for Week 7

Dear God, our wonderful Creator, I pray for my baby's permanent kidneys that are growing this week. I pray for healthy organs, now and all throughout my child's lifetime, that he or she would never experience kidney failure. Let those kidneys function just as they should, filtering out impurities and releasing hormones the body needs.

And, Lord, I also pray for spiritual purity for my baby. Help me, as the mom, and help my child to filter out all the evil that is in this world. Help me teach my child to love what is good and shun what is evil. Protect my child from pornography and from spiritually damaging television, the Internet and movies. Open my spiritual eyes so that I discern what's harmful and keep it out of our home.

Give my child a love for what is righteous and pure and holy. Fill our hearts with so much love for Your Word and for You that we are not drawn into temptation by enticing worldly things. Hebrews 4:12 says that Your Word is alive and powerful and sharper than a two-edged sword; and, Lord, I pray that Your Word will be always in our minds to combat evil. I also ask that You give us Your Holy Spirit to empower us, as You promised in Acts.

In Jesus' name I pray. Amen.

Scriptures for Thought and Meditation

For the word of God is living and effective and sharper than any two-edged sword, penetrating as far as to divide soul, spirit, joints, and marrow; it is a judge of the ideas and thoughts of the heart.
HEBREWS 4:12

The Lord will rescue me from every evil work and bring me safely into His heavenly kingdom.
2 TIMOTHY 4:18

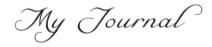

My list of ideas for protecting my child from ungodly influences:

_____

_____

_____

_____

_____

_____

_____

_____

_____

_____

_____

_____

_____

_____

_____

_____

_____

_____

_____

_____

_____

My list of ideas to maintain a godly focus even when I am tired:

_____

_____

_____

_____

_____

_____

_____

_____

_____

_____

_____

_____

_____

_____

_____

_____

_____

_____

_____

_____

8

Tiny Hands and Feet, Fingers and Toes

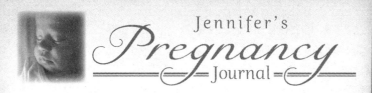

Jennifer's

Pregnancy

Journal

It's the week of Christmas, and I'm feeling pretty emotional. Maybe it's because we're not going to Hawaii to see my family this year. We'll be with Dan's family, and I love them, but it's just not the same.

Christmas is a special time of year for us. Dan loves Christmas more than any other holiday because it represents the birth of our Savior, Jesus. We start decorating in early November, so we have a good six weeks to enjoy the lights and tree before we leave for our vacation around December 15. This year will be a little different, and next year will be even better—we will have a son or daughter to celebrate with!! It will be so amazing to have a little five-month-old to share the joy of Christmas with. I just can't wait! I pray that our son/daughter loves this special holiday as much as we do.

When your baby is born, one of the first things the medical staff does is count the baby's fingers and toes; and every parent does the same. It's a good feeling when you count to 10 and see they're all there. They're so cute! I don't know anybody who doesn't marvel at how exquisite a newborn baby's hands are. Science tells us the fingertips have one of the highest concentration of temperature and touch receptors among all areas of the skin, making them extremely sensitive to heat, cold, moisture, texture, pressure and vibration. Your baby will use these sensory probes to discover the world around him. He will learn to catch a ball, comb his hair, pet a cat and color a picture without consciously maneuvering the fingers. Perhaps you never thought about it before, but when you decide to pick up a mug and pour yourself some coffee, you don't have to think about what your fingers are doing—the movements are involuntary.

Some tasks require conscious effort of the fingers at first, such as playing the piano or typing on a keyboard, until it becomes automatic. I've seen our pianist at church play a song and whisper a message to someone at the same time. Experienced typists can tap out pages without thinking about where their fingers are going.

So many special skills and talents that God gives us involve using the hands and fingers—from rebuilding an engine to creating beautiful calligraphy to decorating a cake. My husband loves to play football, so I know he'll be teaching our kids how to throw a pass. And I'm looking forward to buying a big box of crayons and coloring with my children. We pray that whatever special gifts with which God blesses our baby, these gifts will be used for the glory of the Lord.

When I was pregnant with Micah, I prayed for his hands; I prayed that he would use them to help others and always show love. I prayed that he would cause no harm with his hands; that they would be strong but gentle. I asked God to bless them and use them for His glory, that Micah would make beautiful music for worship and praise. With Malia, I asked for many of the same things. I encourage you to pray for your baby's hands and ask God for what you want for your child.

This week, your baby's feet and toes are also beginning to form. I want my children to walk with Christ all the days of their lives, no matter where their feet take them. I want them to know that Jesus is always with them.

If some of your family members have challenges with their feet, then pray that your baby will not inherit those problems. My mother, on top of hereditary issues, crammed her feet into tight high heels and worked all day in them, because that was the thing to do in

Chicago during the 1960s. And I've had a few problems with my own feet during my pregnancy, and afterward. So I pray against any possible defects that could be hereditary. I don't want my son or daughter to experience the pain of foot problems that I've had.

The elbows and wrists are also developing this week, and your baby may even start flexing them. In addition, your baby's main internal organs continue to grow stronger.

A Mother's Prayer for Week 8

Dear Lord, I pray for my baby's hands and fingers, feet and toes, that they will grow and develop properly. I pray for the elbows and wrists that are developing as well, that they will be good and strong and flex as they should.

Please bless my baby's hands and use them for the good of Your kingdom. Bless my baby's feet and help my child to always walk with You, God.

Lord, I thank You for blessing each one of us with special gifts and talents. I pray that whatever my child does with his or her hands, he or she will do it well and use it for the ministry. Bless the work of my child's hands. Help him to be diligent in his work so he may be viewed to have godly character. And, Lord, bless my child's feet that they might go where You want them to go, for Your ministry.

I know that every good and perfect gift comes from above, and I acknowledge You as our Creator and God. I praise You for all You have done and for all You will do.

In Jesus' name. Amen.

Scriptures for Thought and Meditation

Now as we have many parts in one body, and all the parts do not have the same function, in the same way we who are many are one body in Christ and individually members of one another. According to the grace given to us, we have different gifts.
ROMANS 12:4-6

For when he sees his children, the work of My hands within his,
they will honor My name, they will honor the Holy One of Jacob
and stand in awe of the God of Israel.
ISAIAH 29:23

My Journal

Write a special blessing for your baby. (When your child is old
enough, you can read this together. Be sure to sign and date it.)

_____

_____

_____

_____

_____

_____

_____

_____

_____

_____

_____

Have the father or grandparents write a blessing, and add it here.

_____

_____

_____

_____

_____

_____

_____

_____

_____

_____

_____

9

The Heartbeat of Your Family

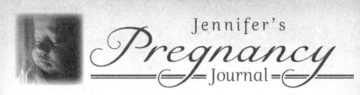

Jennifer's *Pregnancy* Journal

We went to see the doctor this week as a threesome—Dan, myself and two-year-old Micah—and we left confirmed as a foursome. We are pregnant again!

It was especially fun this time, because Micah could see and understand that there was a little baby growing inside of Mommy.

Our eyes were glued to the screen as the technician scanned my tummy; and then, there it was—our tiny baby, just about an inch long. Dan insisted the baby looked just like him!

Micah saw the shape on the screen and asked, "What's that?"

"That is your sister or brother," I said.

The doctor asked Micah if he wanted to hold the heart monitor so that we could all hear the baby's heart beat. That put a huge smile on his face.

"Sure," he said. And then we heard it . . . thump, thump, thump. It seemed so fast, beating to the rhythm of an angelic drummer.

Micah looked amazed. "Wow," he said. Dan kept looking from me to the baby and back to me again. I could see the joy in his eyes. That was a great day.

I was born in Oak Park, Illinois, in 1970, and I had just one sibling at the time, an older sister. Originally, my parents planned on having only two children, but that soon changed.

When I was almost three years old, my parents had enough of the frigid winters and scorching summers in Chicago, so they loaded me, my sister and my new baby brother into a motor home to search for a more desirable place to raise their family. From June until early September, we cruised across 43 states. Although we saw many beautiful sites, including the Rocky Mountains and Grand Canyon, my parents didn't find what they were looking for, so they packed us up again the following summer, and we flew to the South Pacific. We traveled all throughout Tahiti, Samoa, Fiji and Hawaii. We were on 24 flights in three-and-a-half months.

My parents fell in love with Hawaii and liked the fact that it was part of the United States, so they returned to Chicago, sold everything and flew back to Hawaii. Mom and Dad bought a small house overlooking Kailua-Kona Bay and made it into a loving home. We attended a church there on the Big Island of Hawaii called Calvary Community Church.

In spite of my parents' original idea to have just two children, our family grew to nine, including my mom and dad. It always was an exciting time in the house when we were planning for the next baby to arrive. God bestowed my mom with a special gift—mothering!

We had fun and wild times growing up. There was always something going on: a Bible study at our house, a group outing or a church potluck. Now I can look back and see what a truly great life my parents gave us. There were hard times too, but in my heart I always knew that I was loved by my family and by God. The heartbeat of our family was healthy and strong. My parents taught us that talking to God and trusting Him should be part of our daily lives.

We Hear Our Baby's Heartbeat

The day that Dan, Micah and I went to see our second baby's ultrasound, both my husband and I felt the same way—we didn't care if it was a boy or a girl; we just wanted a healthy baby with a good, strong heart. I thought back to growing up in Hawaii in a large family, and I knew there were certain things about the heart of that family that I wanted to carry over into my own family now. A sense of belonging, the way we knew our parents cared for us, and the pursuit of godly ideals—those were all things I wanted for my children too.

When you hear your baby's heartbeat for the first time, I hope you experience God's presence with you and know that you've been blessed with a wonderful gift. And I hope you take some time to think about the heartbeat of your own family and what that means to you. What makes your family special? What bonds you together? How can you invite Jesus Christ to be a central part of your lives?

If it should happen that you don't hear your baby's heartbeat this week, don't panic. It's probably because your baby is snuggling in a cozy corner of your uterus or has his back facing out, making it difficult to pick up the sound. In a week or so, you'll have the joy of hearing the fast-paced *thump-thump* of your baby's heart.

A Mother's Prayer for Week 9

Dear Lord, thank You for this special person growing inside of me. I pray that this time of rejoicing and gladness would also be a time of praising You for Your blessing of the miracle of life. Your Word says that every good and perfect gift comes from above, so I give You my thanks for this wonderful gift.

I pray that my baby grows to be a man or woman after Your own heart. Give him or her a heart for what is right, pure, lovely and good. Help me watch over my baby and bring up my child in a godly way. Help me be an example of Matthew 5:8, where You said, "Blessed are the pure in heart, for they shall see God" (NKJV).

Lord, bond us together as a family. Jesus, we invite You to be the head of our home and central to everything we do. Make us aware of Your presence in our lives on a daily basis. And bless our extended family as well.

If I have any ill feelings toward my parents, I pray that You will help me mend these relationships before my baby comes, or use this baby in a special way to bring us back together. I want this baby to know his grandparents and receive their love as well. Bless us with an extended family.

Lord, I also pray that You develop my baby's heart just perfectly and make it beat in perfect rhythm for all the days of his life. Thank You, Lord, for this special gift. In Jesus' name. Amen.

Scriptures for Thought and Meditation

Test me, LORD, and try me; examine my heart and mind.
PSALM 26:2

The LORD does not look at the things a man looks at. Man looks at the outward appearance, but the LORD looks at the heart.
1 SAMUEL 16:7, *NIV*

My Journal

How I felt when I heard my baby's heartbeat for the first time:

_____
_____
_____
_____
_____
_____
_____
_____
_____
_____
_____

Special things and special times that bond our family together now or will bond us together in the future:

_____

_____

_____

_____

_____

_____

_____

_____

_____

_____

_____

_____

_____

_____

_____

10

Half-a-Million Neurons and Your Baby's Memory

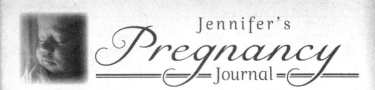

Jennifer's *Pregnancy* ~Journal~

Every night since I found out I am pregnant, I have prayed for my baby; but I never prayed so hard as I did when we got "The Big Scare" this week.

At our last appointment, the doctor informed Dan and me of all the possible risks, birth defects, and so on, and by the time he was done telling us everything that could go wrong, it made Dan feel like it would take a miracle for our baby to be born healthy!

One of the worst experiences of my life was hearing that my baby could be mentally handicapped simply because, like so many moms-to-be, I was above age 35 and therefore automatically considered "high risk." I just hate that term. They don't look at how you eat, exercise or take care of yourself—they only look at your calendar age. I feel healthy, and I know my baby is too. I don't smoke, drink or do drugs; I eat an extremely healthy diet; and I exercise six to seven days a week. I certainly don't feel like I should be in the "high risk" category when I am healthier than many people 10 years younger than me.

The only way I survived "The Big Scare" was through prayer. Thank You, Lord, for hearing my prayer!

"Your baby could have Down's syndrome," said the doctor.

He may as well have shot me with a stun gun. I couldn't move, I couldn't blink my eyes and I couldn't speak.

How could this be happening? We'd waited five years to start our family until we were sure the time was just right. As a certified fitness coach, I was in great physical shape, so this came as a shock. We were overjoyed about being pregnant. I couldn't believe there might be something wrong with our precious little baby.

"I'm going to refer you to a specialist in genetic counseling." He said this like it was the next logical step; but to my mind, there was nothing logical about it. It made no sense whatsoever. I was devastated.

The wait to get in to see the specialist was beyond agonizing. We were terrified. They said we had to wait a whole week, but we just couldn't bear not knowing for that long. My husband called and had a few words of reason with them, and then they managed to squeeze us in after three days.

I knew full well that stress is harmful for the baby, but how does a parent handle being told their child might have something seriously wrong with his brain, which will prevent him from leading a normal life? Somehow, I had to stop my mind from racing through all the "what ifs" and get through this. My developing baby didn't need any stress hormones coming from me.

I prayed every minute of the day. It didn't matter what I was doing, I was praying, praying, praying—pleading with God to bless my unborn baby. "Please, Lord, make him be all right," I cried.

Finally, the day to receive the results came. Dan and I drove all the way downtown, mostly in silence. We were both so scared about the outcome. I tried my best to be positive and upbeat and to exercise faith.

As we walked into the clinic, I barely managed to hold back my tears. They told us to go up to the fourth floor and talk with the genetic counselor. I don't know how fast my heart was beating at that point. Tears kept welling up in my eyes, and I couldn't stop them.

Before we saw the doctor, we had to meet with a genetic counselor. Her job was to go over our family history with a magnifying glass. They were trying to discover if any of the possible problems ran in either of our families. They did not. She then explained that this particular ultrasound I would have could detect more than the previous ones. She asked what we would do if they found conclusive evidence that our baby had spina bifida, a permanently disabling birth defect.

Both Dan and I were adamant that we would keep the baby regardless, and not abort; but we would be open to any corrective measures that might help.

The test was a high-powered ultrasound from which the doctor would be able to tell immediately if the baby had spina bifida or Down's syndrome.

This ultrasound was amazing, because we could see with perfect clarity our baby's body, including arms, legs and head. Our baby was on the move, wiggling and rolling around. The nurse technician said our baby looked healthy, moved in a healthy manner and seemed to be the right size. The heartbeat was good, and all the limbs were the correct measurements for a baby that age. We were starting to feel reassured. Then the doctor came in.

He took one look at my placenta and said, "There's the problem—Swiss cheese placenta!"

The doctor explained that some women have a solid placenta, but mine looked like Swiss cheese with little pools of fluid throughout. He went on to explain that this is also a normal placenta, and it works just fine for the baby; but it does throw out abnormal protein levels into my blood, which explains why the tests came back positive. The end result?

The specialist said, "Your baby is fine. No spina bifida, no Down's syndrome. The weight and size are normal. Everything is normal. Don't worry about a thing!"

I burst into tears. All I could say was, "Thank You, Lord. You've answered my prayers."

Later, we found out that this blood test has a high incidence of error; and in my case, my placenta sent the wrong signals.

In hindsight, I see that this was a time when I grew closer to God. Nonetheless, it was the worst three days of my life. I vowed that if I ever became pregnant again, I would not take that same test. After all, we were going to keep and love the baby no matter what.

The Lord answered my prayers for a healthy baby and carried me through an extremely difficult time during my pregnancy. After that, I continued to pray for our baby every day, determined to harness the power of prayer, as promised in the Bible.

Your Baby's Brain Development and Memory

What's going on at this point in your pregnancy is nothing short of astounding. Your baby's brain is generating 250,000 neurons *each and every minute!* Interestingly, the study of memory in neuroscience reveals two types of memory, which are performed in different regions of the brain:

1. *Procedural memory,* which is related to tasks and can be improved with repetition or practice. This type of memory is used when your baby learns that snuggling him in a certain way means he will soon be fed milk.

2. *Declarative memory,* which involves learning facts, such as telephone numbers. This type of memory is used when your baby learns to memorize and recognize your face and you see that your baby responds to you more than to your friends.

And here's another significant finding: studies have shown that babies react more strongly to sounds they heard while still in their mother's womb than to new sounds introduced after birth. This shows that your baby's memory is already at work! You can use this to your advantage. Remember the story of the woman who read the Bible to her unborn baby throughout her pregnancy? That baby is now a teen who loves God's Word.

When I was pregnant with Micah, I prayed for his brain and memory, and I prayed specifically that God would give him the ability to memorize His Word. It's important for our sons and daughters to have the Scriptures tucked away in their mind, because like Psalm 119:11 says, "Your word have I hidden in my heart, that I might not sin against You" (*NKJV*). As parents, we can't be with our children every moment of every day; but when God's Word is with them, the Holy Spirit will bring it to their memory in times of temptation or difficulty. His Word does not fail to strengthen anyone who has it in memory.

I want to praise God for answering my prayers. God gave Micah the gift to remember Scripture. Micah could recite The Lord's Prayer, Psalm 23 and other Bible verses by the time he was 24 months old. I say this to encourage you to pray specifically for your baby's Scripture memory and then follow up by teaching him or her at an early age. We teach our children the names of colors, animals and the alphabet; it's no harder for them to learn God's Word.

This week your baby officially progresses from being an embryo to a fetus, and congenital abnormalities are unlikely to develop after this week. Here's a tip: If you ever get tempted to worry about your baby's development, turn that energy into positive prayer instead.

So here you are in week 10, and all of your baby's vital organs have been formed and are beginning to work together, according to God's marvelous design. You're one quarter of the way through your pregnancy.

A MOTHER'S PRAYER FOR WEEK 10

Dear Lord,

I pray for my baby's brain development. I pray that my baby will develop a healthy, intelligent brain. And because Your Word says, "Whatever you ask in My name, I will do" (John 14:13), I ask confidently, in faith. I also ask that You will bless my baby with an excellent memory. Lord, help me teach my baby to memorize Scriptures, and help my baby to memorize them easily and quickly.

Psalm 119:11 says, "Your word have I hidden in my heart, that I might not sin against You" (NKJV). I believe it is Your will to hide

Your Word in our hearts, and I ask that for my child. I pray that Bible verses will come to his or her memory quickly in times of need.

I thank You for Your promise of giving us peace, so I don't have to worry about something being wrong with my baby. I declare the power of Your Word and Your Holy Spirit to come to pass. May my baby's brain develop just as it should, and may my child be blessed with a high IQ, to be used for Your glory.

In Jesus' name I pray. Amen.

Scriptures for Thought and Meditation

If only they had such a heart to fear Me and keep all My commands, so that they and their children will prosper forever.
DEUTERONOMY 5:29

For we are glad when we are weak, and you are strong. And this also we pray, that you may be complete.
2 CORINTHIANS 13:9, *NKJV*

My Journal

What I want my baby to remember about me:

_____

_____

_____

_____

_____

_____

_____

_____

_____

_____

What I want my baby to remember about Daddy:

_____

_____

_____

_____

_____

_____

_____

_____

_____

_____

_____

_____

Three of my favorite Bible verses I plan to help my child memorize:

_____

_____

_____

_____

_____

_____

_____

_____

_____

_____

_____

11

Baby Teeth and a Sense of Smell

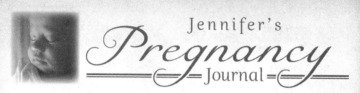

This week was New Year's. I can hardly believe we will have a little one to celebrate the holiday season with next year. It's going to be wonderful.

I'm so grateful for friends and family. Today I really needed to talk with someone who understands what I'm going through. It's weird how my hormones can make me feel so bad some days when this is supposed to be such a beautiful time in my life. I know my husband loves me and he does his best to cheer me up, but he's never been pregnant before. So of course there's no way he can understand exactly what I'm going through.

I talked with my sister, and she gave me her mother-in-law's phone number. She's both a mother and a Christian counselor, so I'll give her a call. I hope she can offer me some words of wisdom.

Don't feel bad if you need to reach out to someone to get perspective on your roller-coaster emotions. God made us to need one another. In fact, Romans 12 talks about how the different parts of our physical body depend on the other parts and compares this to the different members of the Body of Christ depending on one another. During the first trimester especially, changing hormones can take their toll on your energy and emotions. If you're feeling depressed, please find a trusted advisor, such as a Christian counselor, to talk to. Don't try to struggle through your feelings on your own.

God's plans are amazing and wonderful, and this week God's plans for your baby's development include tiny tooth buds growing under the gums. You probably won't see a tooth push through until your child is about six months old; but the start of your baby's teeth is there already.

It was important for me to pray for my baby's teeth during my pregnancy. My own teeth were very crowded together, and I needed braces when I was growing up; but with seven children to support, my parents could not afford them. I believe God answered my prayer, because my son has the most perfect teeth, and I believe his permanent teeth will be good as well. My baby daughter's teeth are just starting to come in, and she's having a hard time with that. I am praying that God will ease the discomfort and help her to be happy. I know that the habit of praying for my children, which I started when they were still in the womb, is a habit I will continue for life. As their mother, I will never stop praying for them—and I am grateful my mother still prays for me.

In week eight, we talked about the hands and fingers, the feet and toes; this week, exquisitely small fingernail and toenail beds begin to develop. Facial development continues and ears take their position. To accommodate all of this development, the blood vessels in your placenta are increasing in order to meet the increasing nutritional needs of your baby.

Your Baby's Sense of Smell

The latest research shows that babies can perceive odors from as early as 11 to 15 weeks. When you think of your sense of smell, what comes to mind? Is it the sweet scent of roses, your grandmother's homemade cinnamon-apple pie, or a baby's skin after a warm bath? Pleasant thoughts come to memory, but God also gave us this sense for our safety. The ability to smell a smoldering fire or detect toxic chemicals can save lives.

What's so amazing about an unborn baby's ability to smell is that he or she doesn't need air or the ability to breathe in order to stimulate the olfactory organ, as previously thought. Now scientists

"Prayer Makes a HUGE Difference!"

Debbie Mills, Senior Prayer Leader for Prenatal Prayer, International House of Prayer

The International House of Prayer is a never-ending, round-the-clock prayer and worship session that's been going since September 19, 1999. Debbie Mills leads the prayer team for women seeking prenatal prayer. Here is part of an interview with my coauthor, Carolyn Warren, on August 26, 2008:

CW: What difference do you think that prayer makes for the expectant mother?

Debbie: Prayer makes a huge difference! The mother has released her fears and is at peace. As a result, her labor is easier and more relaxed. She is focused on the Lord during her labor and delivery. We pray for the mother to have her heart's desire. My granddaughter was born three weeks ago, and my daughter had her at home in a tub of warm water, with only a three-and-a-half-hour labor. That's not for everybody, but it's what she wanted; and the Lord gave it to her.

CW: Congratulations on your new grandchild! That's wonderful. And what difference do you think prayer makes for the baby?

Debbie: Prayer makes a huge difference for the baby, too, because there is so much more peace over the baby—even after the delivery; and the baby is more peaceful in the days that follow.

CW: That's so important. I know that mothers are happy when their babies are peaceful. What other needs do you pray for besides conception?

Debbie: We pray for everything the mother needs. We pray for any fears she has—and we find there are a lot of fears a woman has been carrying that she deals with and releases. We often pray for fear of abandonment. We pray for finances, if that's a concern. Just recently, there was a woman who was going through an adoption, and she came in for prayer. Everything was in order for the adoption to go through, except she was $5,000 short. We prayed for the funds, and within a week, she received a gift of $5,000. Whatever the mother needs, we pray for. We also pray for inner healing to take place. That's important, too.[1]

tell us the amniotic fluid passes through the baby's mouth and nose, triggering the senses of taste and smell.[2]

With all the changes going on at this point, it's no wonder an expectant mom may feel a little overwhelmed on some days!

A MOTHER'S PRAYER FOR WEEK 11

Dear God, I pray for my baby's teeth. You know how important it is to have good, strong teeth and a pleasant smile, and Your Word tells us that when we are concerned with something, You are concerned as well. I ask You to bless my child with good teeth. Help my baby's mouth to form just as it should, and cause the teeth to fit perfectly. And, Lord, thank You for giving us the sense of smell. Please help my baby's perception of aromas develop just the way it should.

And, Lord, I just want to thank You for all the amazing developments that are happening this week inside and outside my baby's body. When I feel tired or overwhelmed, help me remember that You are with me and You strengthen me. Let me experience Your peace with all the changes that are going on in my body, and peace in knowing that You love my baby and are guiding the development according to Your plans.

In Jesus' name. Amen.

Scriptures for Thought and Meditation

Give thanks to the LORD; call on His name; proclaim His deeds among the peoples. Sing to Him; sing praise to Him; tell about all His wonderful works! Honor His holy name; let the hearts of those who seek the LORD rejoice. . . . Give thanks to the LORD, for He is good; His faithful love endures forever.
1 CHRONICLES 16:8-10,34

I can sing to You and not be silent. LORD my God, I will praise You forever.
PSALM 30:12

My Journal

People I can reach out to and count on when I need to talk:

_____

_____

_____

_____

_____

People I can reach out to and count on when I need prayer:

_____

_____

_____

_____

_____

People who can count on me when they need a friend:

_____

_____

_____

_____

_____

How my baby is going to be able to count on me to be there:

_____

_____

_____

_____

_____

Notes
1. To learn how you can visit the prayer room via live webcast, go to www.ihop.org. For more of the interview with Debbie, see chapter 20.
2. "Baby's Development of Senses," by Karin A. Bilich, *American Baby*. http://health.discov ery .com/ centers/pregnancy/americanbaby/senses.html.

12

The Digestive System and Allergies

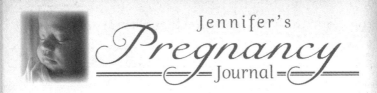

Food has always been a sensitive issue for me since I'm limited on what I can eat due to allergies. I also maintain a healthy eating lifestyle, but during this pregnancy, I've splurged a little. Once in a while is okay for mom and baby.

This week I've been craving lots of bread and pasta. It's really funny, because I was driving past Macaroni Grill the other day, one of our favorite restaurants, and I had never gone in to eat there by myself, but then I thought, why not?

I sat down and the nice waiter brought me a warm loaf of their yummy bread with olive oil and a tall glass of water. My feast began. I ordered a house salad and a dish of angel hair pasta with the meat sauce. I NEVER order pasta, and I rarely eat red meat! But it was so-o-o good! I called Dan to tell him where I was, and I think he got a little jealous.

Your baby is now practicing for when he will eat real food! Quite literally, your baby is flexing his digestive muscle, causing contraction movements. After birth, your child will use this skill to push food through his digestive tract.

Even though the digestive system is developing now, most doctors agree that newborns continue in this development after birth up to the first 13 weeks of life. Also noteworthy: new infants have not yet developed the probiotics that aid digestion. This may explain why some babies are colicky, crying from the discomfort of excess gas trapped in their intestines and bloating in their stomachs. I think it's a good idea to pray for your baby's digestive system during this twelfth week in the womb and on throughout their infancy. I also believe it's important to pray against allergies at this time.

When I was very young, I was allergic to *everything*, from chicken to dairy to dust to animal dander. I was born in Chicago, and the winters there were cold and difficult for me. To keep me warm, my mother dressed me in little stockings, and by the end of the day, my legs would break out from my toes to my hips in a rash similar to eczema.

One day, I was given sherbet in preschool (the teachers didn't realize sherbet had milk in it). They had to rush me to the hospital after I practically stopped breathing. I have photos of myself at about three years old with my stomach so big and bloated from something I ate that I looked like a child from a starving country.

When I was about 10 years of age, I got a puppy, and when I'd bathe her, my arms would break out in hives within two minutes. When I was 12, my eczema spread all over my legs so badly that I could barely walk. All the kids at school teased me about wearing pants on such a hot day—*who wears pants in Hawaii?*

Even as an adult, pets and pollens seem to be the worst allergens for me, and I've spent many sleepless nights in tears because my ears and throat were so itchy I couldn't sleep. Fortunately, I've now outgrown 90 percent of my food allergies, but believe me, I know how awful it is to have allergies. I never wanted my children to go through what I did.

Praying against this matter has touched me deeply. I prayed diligently and consistently while I was pregnant with Micah that he wouldn't inherit allergies from me. I'm so glad we pray to a God who is real and who hears our prayers! To this day, Micah does not have any allergies that we know of.

Some people might wonder if Micah's freedom from allergies was God's doing or simple luck, and there's no scientific way to prove that. But look at it this way: prayer can't hurt, and God's Word supports asking for what we need. John 14:13 says, "Whatever you ask in My name, I will do it so that the Father may be glorified in the Son." John 16:24 says, "Ask and you will receive, that your joy may be complete." Just as we take delight in answering our children's requests, God wants to answer ours; so be encouraged to pray.

A Heart of Compassion

Have you ever thought about how you would handle it if your child is "different"? For myself, having allergies so badly when I was a child made me different. I especially appreciated the people who were compassionate and sensitive to me. These are two Christlike traits to pray for your baby this week.

When I was pregnant, I asked God to give my baby a sensitive and compassionate heart. And you know what? He did. I first began to realize it when Micah was just a baby. He was an extremely happy baby and rarely cried. I remember being at the grocery store one afternoon, and there was a little one crying near us. Micah looked at the baby and got tears in his eyes, and he started crying. It was really sweet, and he's continued to respond to others with sensitivity and compassion many times since then. If he ever sees someone with pain or hurt in their eyes, he asks me what's wrong with the person. He feels their pain.

Throughout the Gospels we see how Jesus showed compassion toward the sick and toward sinners (sparing the woman caught in adultery and dining with the cheating tax collector). Look at what was written by the prophet about Jesus: "The LORD has anointed Me to bring good news to the poor. He has sent Me to heal the broken-hearted, to proclaim liberty to the captives, and freedom to the prisoners" (Isaiah 61:1-2).

Pray that your baby will have those admirable traits too.

A MOTHER'S PRAYER FOR WEEK 12

Dear Lord, this is a special week for my baby. It's the last week of the first trimester and the week in which his digestive system is beginning to develop. Lord, please help my baby develop a strong, healthy system that works in perfect order. I know that many people rely on digestive supplements and over-the-counter medicines to help them in this area, but I pray that my baby will not need anything like that.

And, Jesus, allergies can be life threatening and bothersome. Please allow my baby to be free from any allergies whatsoever. You have the power to do that, and I ask this in Your name.

This week, I'd also ask for Your hand in giving my baby a sensitive and compassionate heart. Help my baby see others in need and to love them like You do. Help my baby to grow up to be a person who brings good news, heals broken hearts and proclaims liberty and freedom to all. Give my child a Christlike attitude toward his family and everyone he meets.

In Jesus' name I pray. Amen.

Scripture for Thought and Meditation

Instead of two Scriptures, I'm listing examples of Jesus' compassion. I encourage you to grab a Bible and look them up, because reading about how Jesus showed compassion in all different kinds of circumstances is a tremendous blessing. Ask the Lord to speak to you as you read His Word.

- Matthew 9:36; 14:14; 15:32; 20:32-34
- Mark 1:41; 3:5; 6:34; 9:25
- Luke 7:12-14,48-50; 10:33-36; 15:1-2
- John 11:33

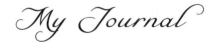

My Journal

I can be a role model for my child in showing sensitivity and compassion to others by:

_____

_____

_____

My thoughts after reading the examples of Jesus showing compassion in all kinds of situations, and knowing that Hebrews 13:8 tells me, "Jesus Christ is the same yesterday, today, and forever."

What I am thinking about my baby today:

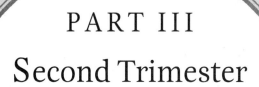

PART III

Second Trimester

WEEKS 13 TO 27

For it was You who created my inward parts;
You knit me together in my mother's womb.
PSALM 139:13

13

Your Baby's Voice

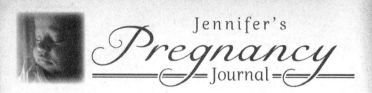

Jennifer's
Pregnancy
Journal

It's been a hard week. I've felt exhausted; and on top of that, Micah has been a handful. I wish I could play with him like I used to, but I just don't have the energy. I want to be Super-Mom; but right now, I'll settle for Okay-Mom.

Yesterday, Micah and I were going to the store when a driver cut us off in traffic, nearly colliding with us. It was scary, because I've got my son and my unborn baby to protect, as well as myself. That incident really tried my patience!

Lord, please give me the endurance, strength and wisdom I need this week. Help me to overcome the temptation to speak angry words when I'm tired and upset, and to speak peace instead.

The Scriptures tell us that our tongue holds the power to speak love, peace and life; or it can speak hatred, criticism and death (see Proverbs 18:21). This week your baby's vocal cords are developing, so you will want to pray that your child will use his or her voice to uplift and encourage people and to glorify God.

According to a psychology study, an 18-month-old child has a speaking vocabulary of 20 words, on average. Just six months later, the vocabulary has grown to 270 words. One year later, at three years of age, the average speaking vocabulary is 900 words. By the time a child is six and ready for first grade, the vocabulary is 2,500 words.[1]

Other studies estimate the average American adult has a vocabulary of 30,000 to 60,000 words. And yet, the English language contains more than 700,000 words.[2] That's a lot of words to use for good or evil!

Some people, like my husband, Dan, use their words to earn a living. When we had been married for just two years, our lives were thrown into a tailspin the day Dan came home from work and could hardly talk.

"What's going on?" I asked him.

"I don't know," he squeaked out in a raspy whisper.

This went on for more than eight months—not good for someone who is a public speaker. We were in a real dilemma.

Dan went to doctor appointment after doctor appointment, but no one knew for sure what caused the trouble. They thought perhaps it was the result of acid reflux, so they put him on a special diet, medication and voice therapy.

None of it worked. You could barely hear him on the telephone.

Finally, Dan got an appointment with a specialist. As we drove downtown, we prayed that this doctor would have some good news.

"Don't worry, God will take care of everything," I said. Dan just smiled.

Dr. Black was very thorough. He explained that he needed to once again run a scope down Dan's nose and into his throat. This procedure is extremely uncomfortable, but it appeared to be the best choice. An intern tried three times without success to get the scope in place, and Dan's white-knuckle grip was getting stronger as he fought to endure. Thank God, the doctor stepped in and said he'd do it.

The doctor said, "You have nodules on your vocal cords, and we will need to do surgery if you ever want to talk again. But you need to understand that there is also a chance you may never speak again."

We were stunned by those words. If Dan lost his voice permanently . . . I'd been joking about how quiet it was in the house lately, because we're both talkers, but I hated the fact that he couldn't talk to me. I've always loved his voice. When we were dating, I used to play his voice messages over and over just to listen to him.

In the car after the appointment with the specialist, we went over each scenario. Dan decided to go ahead with the surgery. He believed that at the rate he was going, his voice would be totally gone sooner or later anyway; and if he didn't do something soon, his business would be seriously harmed. So the surgery was scheduled to take place a few weeks later, and we prayed daily that God would help the surgeon successfully remove the nodules with no permanent damage.

The "big day" finally arrived. After taking Dan to the hospital, I had to train all of my fitness clients and Dan's too.

The hardest thing about this ordeal was that we wouldn't know whether or not it was a success for another 48 hours. We drove home in silence, each with our own thoughts and prayers. We tried to put fear out of our minds as we expected God to do great things through this situation.

Looking back on it now, I can laugh, because every time Dan needed me, he rang a little bell and I jumped up and ran to see what he needed. Then he scribbled on a notepad or he played charades to communicate with me. This went on all weekend.

Sunday morning, our alarm woke us up for church. Still groggy from sleep, out of habit I asked, "What time is it?"

"It's 9:00 A.M.," Dan announced in a totally normal voice— one I hadn't heard for eight months!

With tears in my eyes, I jumped on him and looked at his face. "You can talk! You can talk!" We were both so happy. We lay there and thanked God for giving Dan back his voice.

Words Have Power

Words have the ability to lift up and encourage, or discourage and even bring spiritual death. Psalm 19:14 says, "Let the words of my mouth and the meditation of my heart be acceptable in Your sight, O LORD, my strength and my Redeemer" (NKJV).

It's not too early to pray that your child will reject negative words, such as:

• "I hate myself" or "I hate you."
• "There is no reason to live."

- "I'm not good enough."
- "Nobody cares."

We need to help our children speak positive words by modeling positive speech ourselves, and now is the time to put it into practice and pray toward that end. When you speak a positive message and claim Scriptures through prayer, you release the power of the Holy Spirit to work in your behalf. Pray that your children will use this gift to speak truth and life into every circumstance.

A MOTHER'S PRAYER FOR WEEK 13

Dear Lord,

I pray for my baby's vocal cord development—that his voice will develop properly. Help his mouth, throat, larynx and windpipe to form as they should. And, Lord, I pray that my child will grow up to be a person who is known for speaking words of life. Help my child to speak only positive, encouraging and uplifting words, and to avoid gossip and criticism.

Help me, too, so that I can be a good role model for godly speech. Please help me when I'm having a hard day, when I'm tired or when I'm angry, because I don't want to say things I'll regret later. Help me to hold my tongue. Thank You, Lord, that we can call on You for help.

In Jesus' name. Amen.

Scriptures for Thought and Meditation

May the words of my mouth and the meditation of my heart be acceptable to You, LORD, my rock and my Redeemer.
PSALM 19:14

Pleasant words are a honeycomb: sweet to the taste and healthy to the body.
PROVERBS 16:24

My Journal

My remembrance of a time when someone said something positive that really helped me through a difficult situation:

_____

_____

_____

_____

_____

_____

My remembrance of a time when someone spoke damaging words that hurt me. My thoughts on deciding to forgive the person and experience healing (or deciding not to forgive the person and to hold on to the hurt):

_____

_____

_____

_____

_____

_____

Powerful, positive words from me to my baby today:

_____

_____

_____

_____

_____

_____

Notes

1. "Developmental Psychology Language Development," Uniview Worldwide Ltd. http://www.uniview.co.uk/.../0002%20Language%20Development%20User%20Guide. pdf (accessed November 15, 2009).
2. "Build Your Child's Vocabulary," essortment. http://www.essortment.com/all/build vocabulary_rmuc.htm (accessed November 15, 2009).

14

Your Baby's Legacy

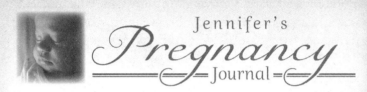

Jennifer's
Pregnancy
—Journal—

I'm so excited! I'm in my second trimester now, and I'm also feeling better. I started taking exercise classes this week; and even though I've taught exercise for years, it's different being a student. I don't have to think about which moves are coming next—I just follow along. And the instructor is great! She was very encouraging about the baby. I'm finding that it is really important to surround myself with supportive, happy, encouraging people.

My mom and I had a good talk on the phone today. I asked her if it was easier raising boys or girls, and she said, "Raising boys and girls is just different, but one isn't harder than the other." That's good to know.

What a fantastic feeling: you've made it to the second trimester! For most women, morning sickness and the risk of miscarrying are now in the past.

By this week, your baby has fully developed sex organs. What's even more amazing is that your baby also has the makings of becoming a parent himself (or herself).

If it's a girl, her ovaries are moving into place. If it's a boy, his prostate is forming now. One day, your child will have the ability to make you a grandparent—and it's already history in the making!

What will your baby inherit from you, and what will your grand-child and great-grandchild inherit from you?

It's remarkable what parents can pass on to their children. Everyone talks about a baby having her father's eyes, her mother's hair or her grandma's long fingers that will surely play the piano someday. But a lot of people don't think about the fact that they can also pass on characteristics like a short temper, a pessimistic outlook or even an unforgiving attitude, especially by their own words and actions. That's why I believe it's important to pray for your unborn baby's future. This week, I want you to pray that he or she will receive a legacy of love, joy, peace, patience, kindness, good-ness, faith, gentleness and self-control (see Galatians 5:22-23).

Don't give in to such negative thoughts as, *I hope my child doesn't get Dad's bad temper,* or *so-and-so's drinking problem.* Instead, claim the characteristics that Galatians 5:22-23 calls the fruit of the Spirit, which is the result of living a life filled with the Holy Spirit. A history of problems in your family tree does *not* mean it is your legacy or your children's legacy. Second Corinthians 5:17 tells us that Jesus came to make all things new. Every individual that names Jesus Christ as their Lord and Savior has the right to put on the righteousness of God in Christ (see 2 Corinthians 5:21).

Colossians 1:12 says, "giving thanks to the Father, who has en-abled you to share in the saints' inheritance in the light." This is your child's legacy. Claim the promises in God's Word for your-self and for your children.

Also happening this week: your baby's thyroid gland that pro-duces hormones and regulates metabolism begins working. The roof of your baby's mouth is formed, and your baby displays a sucking reflex.

A MOTHER'S PRAYER FOR WEEK 14

Dear Lord, I thank You for making it to the second trimester this week! I praise You for the miracle of this baby I'm carrying. Truly, You are a great and wonderful God! I'm amazed at the exquisite detail You planned for Your creation. Thank You for caring for my unborn baby, as You said in so many verses.

Lord, I pray for my child that he or she will exhibit the fruit of the Holy Spirit: love, joy, peace, patience, kindness, goodness, gentleness, longsuffering and temperance. Help me to be a role model of these. Lord, I want to live my life in harmony with You, so that I bring Your Spirit into our home and into my child's life. Help me be the loving mother You want me to be.

And, Lord, I also pray for the physical development of my baby. Please cause everything that is happening this week to develop properly.

Psalm 139:13 says, "You created my inmost being; you knit me together in my mother's womb" (NIV). I thank You for this encouraging Scripture. Please knit together—cause to develop properly—every part of my baby's being: body, soul and spirit.

In Jesus' name. Amen.

Scriptures for Thought and Meditation

He saved us—not by works of righteousness that we had done, but according to His mercy, through the washing of regeneration and renewal by the Holy Spirit. This Spirit He poured out on us abundantly through Jesus Christ our Savior, so that having been justified by His grace, we may become heirs with the hope of eternal life.

TITUS 3:5-7

For you are all sons of God through faith in Christ Jesus. For as many of you as have been baptized into Christ have put on Christ.

GALATIANS 3:26-27

My Journal

The fruit (or characteristics) of the Spirit are love, joy, peace, patience, kindness, goodness, faith, gentleness and self-control. The characteristics I am strongest in are:

_____

_____

_____

_____

_____

_____

The fruit of the Spirit that I want to work on is:

_____

_____

_____

_____

_____

_____

How I will demonstrate the fruit of the Spirit to my child:

_____

_____

_____

_____

_____

_____

The fruit of the Spirit I most want to see in my child:

_____

_____

_____

_____

_____

_____

15

Your Baby's Hair and Skin

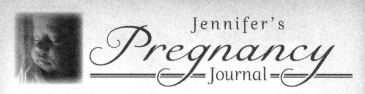

Jennifer's *Pregnancy* Journal

I know why they call the second trimester the honeymoon period of pregnancy. I feel so much better now. I can pretty much eat like normal, and I have my energy back and can almost work out like I used to. Thank You, Lord, for getting me over the hump. There were days when I thought I'd never feel the same.

Dan and I have been doing the spring-cleaning, and he's amazed at the energy I have this week. We have a list of things we want to get done to the house before the baby comes, including fixing up the lower level (or finishing our basement). We're going to put a workout room down there, so it will be convenient for me to work out and train clients with the baby nearby. I'm really looking forward to that.

Your baby's delicate, translucent skin continues to develop, and he or she has a layer of downy-fine hair covering the skin, which protects it before birth.

This week, two tiny eyebrows appear above your baby's eyes. The eyelashes are growing too. I prayed a lot for beautiful eyes with perfect sight for my son, and he has always received comments on how pretty his eyes are and how long his lashes are. Hair is beginning to grow on your baby's head now. It's only the temporary hair at this stage. Some babies are born bald, but most have hair by the time they're six months old. Will your child's hair be curly, wavy or straight? Black, brown, red, blonde or a shade in between? It's fun to think about, but for most families, impossible to predict.

How Your Baby's Hair Type and Color Is Determined

Human hair is controlled by more than one gene. It's not as simple as a child taking after the mother's or father's side. The unknown question is, which parent has the dominant version of the gene?

Every person carries two copies of every gene—one from the mom and one from the dad. Several different genes control the hair, each with two or more versions called alleles. The different versions can combine in unpredictable ways to produce a wide variety of appearances. Hair color is a result of interaction between several genes that control not only color, but also how much pigment ("darkness level") is deposited into the hair shaft. It's all very interesting.

By the time your baby is a teen, he or she will probably have a strong opinion about hairstyle. Remember those days of fussing over hair? As a child grows more independent, the style of his or her hair becomes one way to express individuality and personality. When my niece was a teen, she had gorgeous golden hair down past her waist. Then she cut it all off to her ears and dyed it hot pink! We almost died; but then I thought to myself, *If that's the worst thing my teen ever does, I will be really happy.*

I hope I can help my children to be happy with the hair they're blessed with. Our Malia came out with a little dark brown ponytail, which we all love. But it seems like everyone wants the type of hair they don't have. People with curly hair want to straighten it, and people with straight hair work at making it wavy or curly. Personally, I have dark brown hair, but I'd like it lighter.

Your Baby's Skin Tone

Speaking of inheriting traits from parents and grandparents, genetic scientists tell us that skin color is probably the most complex of all physical traits. According to the latest estimates, there are about six genes that determine skin color; and since we have two copies of each gene (one each from mom and dad), there are 12 possible contributions to the skin color trait. This means that your baby can have from 0 to 12 genes that give varying dosages of color. Your baby randomly receives half (six) genes from you and six from your husband. It's like a beautiful, complex puzzle created by God. And only He knows in advance what your baby's skin tone will look like.

Your baby's skin will do more than make him or her look beautiful. The skin is the body's largest organ, and it functions in four ways:

1. It helps regulate body temperature.
2. It protects the internal organs from physical and chemical injury.
3. It protects the body from invasion of microorganisms.
4. It synthesizes vitamin D, which is diffused into the blood vessels. (Infants and children who lack vitamin D can get a bone malady called rickets.)

While growing up in Hawaii, I always wanted to be like the local people and have dark skin. My girlfriends and I would lie in the sun for hours to get a tan. We'd try to see who could get her face to peel off like a mask. Of course, we regret it now. I am teaching my children how to protect their skin from harmful things like too much sun exposure, and I'm praying for their good health.

Let's also pray that your child will be content with the way God made him or her. First Timothy 6:6 says, "But godliness with contentment is a great gain."

A MOTHER'S PRAYER FOR WEEK 15

Dear Lord, I pray for my baby's hair and skin. Thank You for the wonderful way You make us, with hair to beautify our appearance. I pray that as my child grows, she will be pleased with the type of hair You've given her. Help me instill a healthy self-esteem in my child, so she grows to be a happy person, content with the way she looks but not vain or narcissistic.

I pray for my baby's skin, that it will be healthy and perform the functions You've created it to do. Thank You for giving us beauty combined with protection in the organ that is our skin.

You are a wonderful, loving God. Your Word says that You even know the number of hairs on our head, and I know that means You are concerned with every detail of us. Thank You for caring and loving us so much. I praise You for my baby, growing inside me. I know that You love my baby and see her even as she is yet unborn.
In Jesus' name. Amen.

Scriptures for Thought and Meditation

But even the hairs of your head have all been counted. Don't be afraid therefore . . .
MATTHEW 10:30-31

Casting all your care upon Him, because He cares about you.
1 PETER 5:7

My Journal

A funny or interesting story about my hair to share with my child:

_____

_____

_____

_____

_____

_____

_____

_____

_____

_____

_____

_____

_____

_____

My struggles in being content with my appearance when I was a child and teenager:

_____

_____

_____

_____

_____

_____

_____

_____

_____

_____

_____

_____

My thoughts on how I can help instill in my child a good sense of self-esteem about his or her appearance:

_____

_____

_____

_____

_____

_____

_____

_____

_____

_____

_____

_____

16

Your Baby's Future Mate

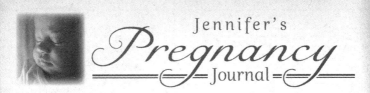

Jennifer's *Pregnancy* Journal

My little one must really be growing, because my appetite has increased! Sometimes I don't feel pregnant, but I know I am, and I think about it constantly, pretty much 24/7. It's hard to concentrate on anything else. All I've been doing is dreaming about meeting my little baby. These nine months are going by really slow!

We started on the baby's room this week, which was a lot of fun. I'm painting a jungle/animal theme all around the room, and my girlfriends are going to help. I found this super cute bedding set, and we're going to copy and enlarge the animals onto the walls. Because we don't know if the baby is going to be a boy or girl, this should work either way. I can't wait to see the room when it's done.

I hope this baby likes jungle animals!

If you could observe your baby's face right now, you'd see a variety of expressions. Yes, your baby's facial features and muscles are developed enough for him to frown, smirk and grin. It would be cute if he were frowning when he heard you say you don't feel well and grinning when he thought about coming out and meeting you; but we know that's not the case. At this point, facial expressions aren't related to any thoughts or emotions.

Your baby continues to grow and is now about three ounces and between four and five inches long. No wonder you're hungry!

But remember, you need only 300 extra calories a day to support your tiny baby's growth.

If you're having a girl, here's a mind-boggling fact: this week, *millions* of eggs are forming in her ovaries. God has already planned your future grandchildren!

It's amazing to think that someday I will be a grandma, or *tutu*, as they say in Hawaii. I honestly never thought about it until I had my own children and my mom became a grandma to them. My children actually have three sets of grandparents who all shower them with love. It's a special relationship between these grandparents and my children, and my prayer is that I can be there when Micah and Malia have their children.

My deepest desire and prayer for my children is that they will follow after God, and He will be the one to write the story of their lives. I pray that they will know God and love Him more than anything else.

I hope that when Micah and Malia are grown and have families of their own, we can all live close by so that I can see them often, help out with baby-sitting, and enjoy my grandchildren as they grow up. I hope that I may bring some form of wisdom and joy their way.

It's never too soon to pray about future events. I began praying for Micah's wife while I was still pregnant with him, because I want him to someday have the perfect partner, picked out by God, just for him. While waiting for Micah's birth, I prayed for this little girl, who is probably not even born yet, and for her parents. I prayed that they know and love the Lord and will raise her in a loving Christian home. I prayed for wisdom, beauty, grace and love to be strong in my future daughter-in-law; and that we will have a special and close relationship.

And for Malia, I pray for her future husband. I pray that he is a man of God, a wonderful communicator and someone who will treat her with love and respect. I pray that he will be a good, loving father and that we all will get along well—since I plan on living close by!

While we're on the subject of praying about your child's future, I want to remind you of the power of words and how you can speak life through the act of blessing your unborn child and then continuing to speak that blessing as he or she grows up. You will want to say things to your baby like, "May you grow up to be a man after

God's own heart" or "May you be a woman who loves the Lord your God with all your heart, soul, mind and strength."

An equally significant way to affect your child's destiny is to pray God's Word over your baby as a way of affirming God's care and His faithfulness to His promises. Choose a Scripture verse or passage you will use as a special daily prayer for your unborn child. For example: "I pray that you may live a life worthy of the Lord and may please Him in every way" (Colossians 1:10). It's okay to paraphrase Scripture to personalize it. Here is an example from Proverbs 31 for a daughter: "I pray that you will speak with wisdom, and that faithful instruction will be on your tongue. I pray that you will watch over the affairs of your household . . . that your children will arise and call you blessed; that your husband will do the same, and he will praise you" (Proverbs 31:26-28, paraphrased).

There are so many biblical prayers and blessings in the Bible for you to search out and choose for your child. (If you'd like to read more examples, take a look at the apostle Paul's beginning words in each of his letters to the Galatians, the Ephesians, the Philippians and the Colossians; or check out the spiritual armor passage in Ephesians 6, beginning with verse 10. And don't forget scriptural blessings like the one found in Jude, vv. 24-25.)

This week, pray for your baby's growth and for his or her future mate. Choose a special Scripture to pray over your unborn baby, and a blessing to say to him or her every day. This is intercessory prayer—standing in the gap for someone else as a link between earth and heaven. What a privilege it is to be in partnership with the Lord for your child in this way.

Remember Psalm 139:13: "For it was You who created my inward parts; You knit me together in my mother's womb."

A MOTHER'S PRAYER FOR WEEK 16

Dear Lord, I pray for my baby's growth. As his or her face continues to develop, please cause everything to come together to form a beautiful child.

If I'm having a girl, I pray for her ovaries and eggs that will give her children someday. Lord, Your plans are so awesome. Your Word says that children are an inheritance from the Lord, and I pray that my daughter will have the blessing of being a mother one day. And, God, I pray for my daughter's future husband, that You will bring a good, kind, loving, wise man into her life; and most of all, that he will be a man of God who loves You and follows Your Word.

If I'm having a boy, I pray for my son's future wife. Bless her and bring her and my son together in Your timing. I pray that she will be a woman who loves my son and is a good and faithful wife; but most of all, that she is a woman of God who loves You and follows Your Word.

Lord, You said that You delight in giving us the desires of our heart, so I ask that I will have a special, loving relationship with the mates of my children, that we will all get along and enjoy one another's company. I also ask for the blessing of being an integral part of my grandchildren's lives to help them, to pass on wisdom and to be a blessing to them.

In Jesus' name. Amen.

Scriptures for Thought and Meditation

Sons are indeed a heritage from the LORD, children, a reward.
PSALM 127:3

I have no greater joy than this: to hear that my children are walking in the truth.
3 JOHN 4

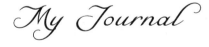

A special Scripture verse or passage I have chosen and personalized for my unborn baby and will pray for him (or her) every day:

_____

_____

_____

_____
_____
_____
_____
_____
_____

A blessing based on godly character qualities that I will speak out loud to my unborn baby before I go to sleep at night, and continue to speak to my baby after he or she is born:

_____
_____
_____
_____
_____
_____
_____
_____
_____

Advice I will give my children early on about what is most important to seek in the person they eventually will choose to marry:

_____
_____
_____
_____
_____
_____
_____
_____
_____

17

Your Baby's Body Fat and Self-Image

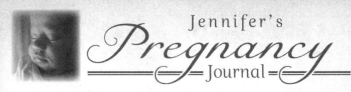

Jennifer's *Pregnancy* Journal

We found a crib and changing table at a sale for cheap. I know we probably won't use the crib right away, because I'm going to nurse the baby, and I want him (I still think it's a boy) right close to me and at arm's reach. I don't want to have to get out of bed multiple times a night to feed him. My mom kept us in bed with her, and I'm going to follow her tradition. I think it makes for a happier baby. Just my opinion, and I know it's not for everyone.

This little one has been kicking a lot, directly under my right breast; he must have a foot or hand that keeps pushing on my rib all day long. I have to use my hand to physically move it away, because sometimes it really hurts.

Your baby is gaining body fat this week, plumping up, and will continue to do so until she or he is born. This is a good thing, as long as your baby is adding the normal, essential layers of fat that are necessary for keeping the baby warm after his or her entrance into the world. But in our modern American culture, too often unborn babies are forced into obesity by mothers who eat double and triple the calories they need to support their pregnancy. An overweight newborn is disadvantaged from the get-go, because he or she is at risk for acquiring obesity-related health problems.

We live in a society that puts a tremendous amount of value on being slim and attractive, so it's no wonder that so many people have an issue with self-image and body weight. I was affected by this myself.

Growing up in a large family in Kailua-Kona, Hawaii, we spent a lot of time enjoying the outdoors, and we led an active lifestyle. But then I went away to college in California, and so many things changed. Like a lot of college girls, I gained the "freshman forty"—and I'm only 5′ 2″, so that was a lot.

When someone in Hawaii who hadn't seen me while I was away saw me again, he looked at me and said, "What the heck happened to *you?*" That didn't make me feel very good!

So, I decided right then and there to make a change.

I became involved in fitness training and lost 42 pounds in six months. I loved fitness training so much that I went on to become a Certified Fitness Trainer and Nutrition Expert.

Ten years later, I met my wonderful husband, who was also a fitness trainer.

As you can imagine, the last thing in the world I wanted to do when I became pregnant was to gain a lot of extra weight and go back to how I was while I was in college. So weight gain and health are both important issues for me. I studied and worked hard to gain only a healthy amount of weight and to have a healthy pregnancy and healthy baby. Now I do my best to use my experience to be a blessing to other moms-to-be by coaching and providing information to them too. (If you'd like to find out more, please visit me at www.PrayForYourBaby.com.)

One thing I want for my children, and especially for my daughter, Malia, is to have a healthy self-image and to be happy with her body. I don't want her to compare herself to worldly celebrities or anorexic models. I want her to be healthy, to feel good about herself and know that her parents and God love her very much just as she is. The same thing applies to our son, Micah. Dan and I are committed to that, and we believe that living healthy is part of presenting a good testimony for the Good News of Jesus Christ. So this week, I want you to pray that your unborn baby will gain a healthy amount of body fat and have a healthy self-image. And then for the future, pray that your baby will develop inner beauty that is lasting and forever. It's never too soon to pray for your child's self-esteem and body image. Our children definitely need our prayer support. As 1 Peter 3:3-4 says, "Your beauty . . . should consist of the hidden person of the heart with the imperishable quality of a gentle and quiet spirit, which is very valuable in God's eyes."

A Mother Proclaims Scripture for Her Daughter's Breakthrough

Beverly McIntyre is a mother who, through prayer, became her daughter's source of healing when she was suffering from a poor self-image and bulimia and anorexia. Beverly says, "Draw a line in the sand and tell Satan he can't cross over it, because God has given you the authority to fight in His name. Become a prayer weapon for God until that child experientially walks in the victory of Isaiah 54:13: "All your children shall be taught by the LORD, and great shall be the peace of your children" (NKJV).

Beverly walked the halls of the hospital where her daughter was behind locked doors battling bulimia and anorexia, praying and proclaiming Isaiah 54.

She goes on to say, "No one will ever love your child as much as you do. You are the one who is called to pay the price in prayer. Find a Scripture and stand upon its truth until the Lord gives you the assurance that the breakthrough happened."[1]

You can read her story of intercessory prayer and victory for her daughter in the magnificent book *Intercessors: Discover Your Prayer Power* by Elizabeth Alves, Tommi Femrite and Karen Kaufman.

A MOTHER'S PRAYER FOR WEEK 17

Dear Lord, as my baby continues to grow, I pray that she will gain the right amount of weight, including the healthy amount of body fat. Please help me to eat in a healthy way and exercise on a regular basis so I don't put my baby in jeopardy of having diabetes or other obesity-related health issues. Give me the strength to avoid junk foods and excessive sugar and fat.

Lord, help me to concentrate on good health and not become obsessed with body weight and body image. I know my self-worth comes from You, and not from the way I look. Please help me with that, and help me pass on to my child only good attitudes about her appearance and her weight. Protect my child from eating disorders and a poor self-image.

Empower us, as a family, to live a healthy lifestyle. Empower us to be good testimonies of Your love, forgiveness and life-changing power. I pray that we would shine from an inner glow of Your Holy Spirit, and that it would attract people to You.

Dear God, please continue to bless and guide my baby's development. I thank You for Your love and protection.

In Jesus' name. Amen.

Scriptures for Thought and Meditation

*Do you not know that your body is the sanctuary
of the Holy Spirit who is in you, whom you have from God?
You are not your own, for you were bought at a price;
therefore glorify God in your body.*
1 CORINTHIANS 6:19-20

*Your beauty should not consist of outward things like
elaborate hairstyles and the wearing of gold
ornaments or fine clothes; instead, it should consist of
the hidden person of the heart with the imperishable
quality of a gentle and quiet spirit, which are
very valuable in God's eyes.*
1 PETER 3:3-4

My Journal

I will help my child feel good about the way she/he looks by:

_____

_____

_____

_____

_____

_____

_____

_____

_____

_____

I will help my child understand that inner beauty is the most important type of beauty by:

_____

_____

_____

_____

_____

_____

_____

_____

_____

_____

Note

1. Elizabeth Alves, Tommi Femrite, Karen Kaufman, *Intercessors: Discover Your Prayer Power* (Ventura, CA: Regal Books, 2000), pp. 31-34.

18

Are You Having a Boy or a Girl?

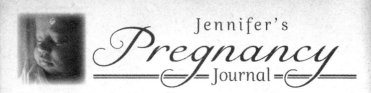

Jennifer's
Pregnancy
Journal

During my pregnancy with Micah, I always felt I was going to have a boy. (And I was right!) Now pregnant for the second time, I feel like this one is going to be a girl. Dan thinks it's another boy, but he was wrong the first time, so . . . we'll see.

I love having a boy and would really love another one. Micah would just love to have a brother to play with. But having a daughter would be special too. My mother says the great thing about having a daughter is that she keeps in touch more. Once a son gets married, he doesn't call as much or visit as often. On the other hand, with a daughter, once she gets married, she calls all the time to talk about her husband, her pregnancy and her kids . . . I think she was referring to me!

If you're having a girl, her uterus and fallopian tubes are developed by the end of this week. And if you're having a boy, his prostate and genitals are developing now. I'm reminded of Genesis 1:27:

> So God created man in His own image;
> He created him in the image of God;
> He created them male and female.

What a marvelous message from God, that He designed us to be in His own image, able to communicate with Him, and to be male or female—both His design!

During my pregnancies and even continuing on now, I pray for my son and daughter to celebrate how God made them, and yet to exercise sexual purity. In this age of sexual exhibitionism and exploitation, it's a great challenge for our young people to stay sexually pure until marriage. Teens are bombarded with sexual messages, and I pray for my children to hold on to God's Word and have the strength to say no to temptation. It might not be popular, but following God's way of abstinence saves a lot of heartache and, oftentimes, disaster. I'm sure we all know young men and women who have been hurt by becoming sexually active before marriage.

When you read my Christian testimony in Appendix 2, you will find out that I was one of those teens. I learned the hard way, and now I pray that my children do not engage in premarital sex. First Peter 2:11 says, "to abstain from fleshly desires that war against you." There are so many things that can happen when a person has sex outside of marriage: abortion, sexually transmitted diseases, AIDS and having a child too early.

Someone very close to me got pregnant when she was 15. I remember feeling stunned when I found out; I just couldn't believe it. As a result, she had to drop out of high school to try to raise a child on her own.

She had a lot of voices around her telling her to abort the baby or give it up for adoption, so it was a confusing time for her. Thank God she had Christian parents and friends who didn't judge her but reached out in compassion to help her instead. The end of this story is a happy one. Her circle of support helped her to raise a wonderful daughter and send her to a Christian school, where she became the valedictorian of her graduating class.

As parents, we want and hope for the best for our children. We teach them and pray for them that they will overcome temptation and wait until they get married to have sexual relations. So this week, not judging or condemning anyone at all, I want you to pray for your children to value sexual purity and follow God's way.

A Mother's Prayer for Week 18

Dear Lord, I pray for the sexual development that's going on in my baby's body. I thank You that You made us so wonderfully, and I pray that my baby's body and hormones will develop properly, just as You designed.

And, Lord, I pray for sexual purity for my child. Help me to teach my child to follow Your ways, and give me wisdom to answer tough questions. Help me keep a watch over my child and protect him or her, as a godly parent should. Make my child strong against temptation and the pull of the world. I pray that he or she will not sacrifice godly principles for popularity. Instill Scriptures in his or her heart so that he or she does not sin against You, as Proverbs 119:11 says. Protect my family and keep us under the shelter of Your Holy Spirit.

In Jesus' name. Amen.

Scriptures for Thought and Meditation

But now God has placed the parts, each one of them, in the body just as He wanted.
1 CORINTHIANS 12:18

I have treasured Your word in my heart so that I may not sin against You.
PSALM 119:11

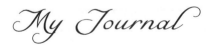

Thoughts and wisdom to share with my child someday on how a desire for popularity or love can lead to actions that could affect his/her life in a negative way (include sexuality, but think beyond that):

_____

_____

_____

_____

_____

_____
_____
_____
_____
_____
_____
_____

My thoughts on how I can equip my child to choose sexual purity, until marriage, in a less than pure world where he/she will be bombarded with impure messages (think in terms of developing your child's critical thinking skills):

_____
_____
_____
_____
_____
_____
_____
_____
_____
_____
_____
_____
_____

19

Your Baby Strikes a Pose

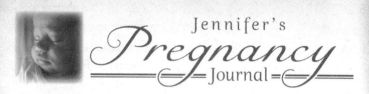

Jennifer's *Pregnancy* Journal

I heard a tragic story today. One of my friends has a friend who was expecting a baby, and tests indicated that her baby had Down's syndrome. Her husband wanted to terminate the pregnancy; of course, the mother did not. This caused such a conflict between them that they ended up getting divorced. The woman went on to have the baby by herself, and the baby was born perfectly, 100 percent normal. How sad. The false results of the test really messed up their lives.

I'm thankful that Dan and I were in agreement and prayed together when we got our "Big Scare." If I have another baby, I'll never do that blood test again. The stress it put on my body was awful and, in the end, it provided no benefit.

Please don't take my journal entries the wrong way. Every pregnancy is different. Your body is unique, and each baby develops at a different pace. I would never presume to tell another mom-to-be whether or not she should take a certain test; that's between you, your doctor and God. So pray about it and make the choice that's right for you.

You might get some clues about your baby's personality this week. Do you have a content, peaceful child who smiles, yawns and has a long, leisurely stretch? Or do you have a real go-getter, doing flips and somersaults? Get ready, because your baby is capable of performing a lot of action this week and from this point on. I think it's got to be one of the most awesome experiences to feel a growing baby inside of you, moving.

I remember the first time I felt "something." It can be almost like you're not sure if it's the baby or just gas. But then you feel it again—and then you know, someone else is a part of you.

One time, while we were in Hawaii visiting my parents, when I was pregnant with Micah, Dan and I were at the pool. I looked over and saw Dan staring at my tummy and laughing. He couldn't believe what he was seeing. My whole stomach was lurching right and left, like it was doing the cha-cha. He thought a hand or foot was going to poke out at any minute!

Up to this week, your baby has had his legs curled and tucked under, but now he's straightened out his legs. You might feel some dancing or gymnastics going on in there! And did you know that on ultrasound images, they've even seen babies open their mouth and stick out their tongue?

Take a look at all the things your baby can do when he or she is not sleeping:

· smile and frown	· hiccup	· rotate	· open his mouth and
· suck and swallow	· breathe	· lift his head	stick out his tongue
	· yawn	· flip	
	· stretch	· somersault	

Yes, you've got a dynamic person with his or her own unique personality already being acted out inside of you. A story came to us from an employee at a pregnancy counseling center, who wants to remain anonymous. But Carolyn Warren was privileged to have a face-to-face interview with her. Here's what happened.

A young woman entered the counseling center with her boyfriend. The boyfriend was putting a lot of pressure on her to end her pregnancy because he was afraid of how her mother would react when she found out he'd gotten her daughter pregnant. He was ashamed of violating the mother's trust and didn't want to fall out of her good graces. He thought it would be better to just end the pregnancy.

Unbeknownst to this young couple, the staff at the counseling center had just spent the morning praying that God would miraculously touch whoever walked through the doors that day.

Because the young woman was 13 weeks pregnant, she was set up with the staff nurse to perform an ultrasound, which was routine for health precautions.

As she was performing the ultrasound, suddenly the nurse exclaimed, "This is astonishing! In the many hundreds of ultrasounds I've performed over the years, I've never seen this before."

The girlfriend peered at the monitor for a closer look as the nurse said, "Look here, the baby is lounging with his hands behind his head!"

Just then she looked up to see that her boyfriend was standing with his hands behind his head in the exact position of his unborn son. This was his "signature posture," one he used all the time.

When the boyfriend saw the replica of himself on the screen, he shouted, "That's OUR KID! Honey, we're going to keep this baby. We'll go talk to your mom together, tonight."

As the staff member relayed this story, tears formed in her eyes. God had answered their prayers by showing the unborn baby's personality to the father at just the right time when an ultrasound could capture his movements; it had saved his life.

Who knows what cute signature moves your baby may be making now, while he or she is growing inside you? Well, don't worry; soon you'll get to see those moves every day, because you're almost halfway to your delivery date. This week, I want you to pray not only for your baby's growth, but also for his or her personality—what I call the "happiness factor." Whether you have a thoughtful, quiet introvert or a rambunctious extrovert, I think that as mothers what we want most is for our children to know the love of God and to be happy.

A Mother's Prayer for Week 19

Dear Lord, I praise You for this wonderful life growing inside of me. I pray that my baby will continue to grow properly and be 100 percent healthy. Cause all the parts of the body to grow right and be strong. And, Lord, I pray that my child will have a happy heart and joyful spirit. Give him or her a personality that draws others to want to be friends.

Lord, please make all of my test results accurate and with a good result. Give the doctors wisdom. If anything is amiss at this point, heal my baby and make him totally, completely perfect, in Jesus' name. I stand on the holy Bible that promises us that God heals ALL diseases. You are our Creator and Healer, Lord God, and I claim perfect health for my baby.

God, You are awesome, and I thank You for the miracle of this baby growing inside of me. Please help this entire pregnancy to go smoothly, and help me to enjoy this amazing time in my life. This truly is a gift from You, and I praise You for it.

Thank You, Lord. In Jesus' name. Amen.

Scriptures for Thought and Action

You are my hiding place; You protect me from trouble.
PSALM 32:7

The one who lives under the protection of the Most High dwells in the shadow of the Almighty. I will say to the LORD, "My refuge and my fortress, my God, in whom I trust."
PSALM 91:1-2

My Journal

My doctor has done the following tests, and the results were:

_____

_____

_____

_____

_____

_____

_____
_____
_____
_____
_____
_____
_____
_____

I will have no fear because:

_____
_____
_____
_____
_____
_____
_____
_____
_____
_____
_____
_____
_____
_____
_____

20

Your Baby's Special Moisturizer

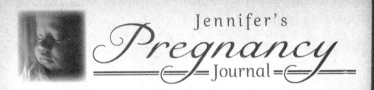

Jennifer's *Pregnancy* Journal

The weather is finally getting better! I'm such a Kona girl at heart; I just hate the snow and cold. I'm getting outdoors a lot more now, and I'm loving the fresh air. I feel so much healthier when I'm in the sun a little. I can't wait for summer!

This little one has been kicking more lately, which wakes me up. But what's more difficult is that my neck and back have been bothering me. I wake up around 3:00 or 4:00 in the morning, and then I can't fall back asleep for hours. I know this is the beginning of the end for getting eight hours of uninterrupted rest. I can't help but feel like this is God's way of getting me ready for those nighttime feedings.

Not every day is easy—but I'm officially halfway there—and that counts for something!

Good news! Week 20 is the official halfway point on the 40-week pregnancy calendar. It feels great to know that approximately half of your pregnancy is behind you!

To encourage your faith, I have another story about how God answered prayer for a young couple who wanted a baby. Betsy Leeuwner of Phoenix, Arizona, had been trying to get pregnant for more than four years. She had the disappointment of a miscarriage, but no successful pregnancy.

Unbeknownst to her, one Sunday morning at New Heart Worship Center in Auburn, Washington, Betsy's mother, Jo Lembo, responded to a call from God. Senior Pastor Gordon Banks felt led of the Holy Spirit to invite couples that wanted a baby but had been unable to get pregnant to come forward to the altar for prayer. By faith, Jo went forward to stand for her daughter Betsy, who lived three states away.

Just weeks later, Betsy got pregnant. Mr. and Mrs. Leeuwner made the happy announcement that they were expecting a baby, and both they and the grandparents-to-be are praising God for answered prayer.

God Watches Over Your Baby

Just think, if God answers prayer for the conception of a baby, don't you think He also answers prayers for the baby's health and development? Of course, He does.

The great American evangelist Billy Graham said, "Heaven is full of answers to prayers for which no one ever bothered to ask." I, for one, don't want to be guilty of not asking God for everything my baby needs.

The main event in your baby's development this week is the velvety soft skin. It is separating into the four layers of the epidermis; and the skin for the palms and bottoms of the feet is forming as well.

Remarkably, a protective layer of creamy white moisturizer, called the vernix, covers your baby's skin this week while it's developing.[1] This is no cheap drugstore product—this natural emollient performs multiple functions, such as the following:

- It protects your baby's skin from scratches.
- It contains the antioxidants vitamin-E and melanin to help the baby's skin cope with the baby's entry into air at birth.
- It has anti-infective property to protect from bacterial invasion.
- It hydrates the skin, being made of 80 percent water.
- It may help regulate temperature of the skin.

Interview with Debbie Mills

Prayer Leader for Prenatal Prayer,
International House of Prayer (IHOP)

CW: Does IHOP have regular prayer for couples that are trying to conceive?

Debbie: Yes, we pray three times a week for women who want to get pregnant, as well as for those who are going through their pregnancy. We have women come from all over the world.

CW: Can you tell me how that works?

Debbie: They come into the prayer room and sit in the back. We then cover them with "soaking prayer"; that is where we pray silently for them. Then three prayer ministers pray for each individual. One leads the prayer, and the others intercede. We intercede for the woman's needs and we pray the Scriptures and call forth the gifting for the baby. We're seeing wonderful things happen. For example, a woman who had traveled from Illinois for prayer came running into the room from the back; she was just ecstatic, and she screamed, "I was barren for seven years, and I'M PREGNANT!"

CW: Praise God, that's wonderful! How is the prayer room at IHOP set up?

Debbie: Prayer and worship go on 24 hours a day, 7 days a week. We have full worship teams consisting of singers and those who play musical instruments. The teams switch out every two hours. When you're there praying, you don't even notice the switch; you might just look up after a while and see there is a new worship group ministering. So it's a combination of worship and intercession. Our model is from King David, who brought in people to minister in the tabernacle (see 1 Chronicles 22–24). If women who want prayer can come visit us, then that would be great. If not, they can view the prayer room and pray from home, using their computer, by logging on to www.ihop.org.[2]

I was thinking about this extra-fancy moisturizer that protects the unborn baby, and it made me think about how good God is to watch out for every need we have. If God made your baby's oil gland to produce vernix, don't you think He cares about watching over all of your baby's health? Absolutely.

A MOTHER'S PRAYER FOR WEEK 20

Dear Lord,

I thank You for hearing and answering my prayers. Your Word tells us that You are touched by our feelings, and that You care for us. And, Jesus, You showed how much You love the little children when You took them in Your arms and blessed them. So this week, I am praying to thank You that I've made it to the halfway point on the pregnancy calendar, and I pray for my baby's continued growth and development.

It is so awesome the way You designed pregnancy to take care of the baby's needs. I pray for my baby's skin as it is growing the four layers this week. Help the moisturizing vernix to be produced and do its job. Protect my baby's skin from scratches, dehydration and infection. When my baby is born, protect the skin from harm.

Protect my baby, both physically and spiritually. Keep my child safe in Your loving arms. In the name of Jesus. Amen.

Scriptures for Thought and Meditation

Rejoice in hope; be patient in affliction;
be persistent in prayer.
ROMANS 12:12

Devote yourselves to prayer;
stay alert in it with thanksgiving.
COLOSSIANS 4:2

My Journal

How I feel about being halfway through my pregnancy:

_____

_____

_____

_____

_____

_____

_____

_____

_____

_____

How my expectations have increased and/or changed:

_____

_____

_____

_____

_____

_____

_____

_____

_____

_____

_____

Notes

1. Gurcharan Singh and G. Archana, "Unraveling the Mystery of Vernix Caseosa," *Indian Journal of Dermatology,* 2008, vol. 53, pp. 54-60.
2. To read a birth story from IHOP, see chapter 28.

21

Strong, Healthy Bones

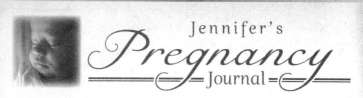

Dear Baby,
I don't know you yet, but I love you already. You will be born in July, and we can't wait to meet you, Micah or Malia. I pray for you every day, every night, and all of the time. I pray that you will be happy, healthy, loving, joyful, wise and beautiful on the inside and out. I know you will come out just perfect.

I am also praying that your daddy and I will be good parents to you. We love you already!
Love,
Mommy and Daddy

The big news this week is that your baby's bone marrow—that flexible tissue inside the bones—is developed enough to produce blood cells.

All blood cells are produced in the bone marrow, and most of a child's bones produce blood, which carries nutrients to every part of the body and then takes away the waste again.

It's important to have strong bones, both while growing up and growing older. I grew up in a home where several people in the family had an allergy to dairy products, so we never had cow's milk in the house. To make sure we got enough calcium, every morning my father stirred calcium powder into our oatmeal, along with some honey. I grew up drinking goat's milk, almond milk or rice milk. And even though I've outgrown my milk allergy, I still use the delicious almond milk to make protein shakes at home for Micah and myself.

The National Institutes of Health says that 99 percent of our body's total calcium is stored in our bones and teeth. When you're pregnant or breastfeeding, you need 1,200 mg of calcium each day. I recommend taking supplements that contain calcium along with magnesium and Vitamin D to aid with calcium absorption; in addition, other good sources of calcium are low-fat yogurt, cheddar cheese, milk, cottage cheese, kale and broccoli.

Because I'm a personal trainer, women often ask me if it's okay to do weight-bearing exercises during pregnancy. The answer is yes, as long as you lift the proper amount of weight for your fitness level and for your stage of pregnancy, and in the correct way. Exercising with weights benefits you in five ways:

1. Helps strengthen your bones and muscles
2. Improves your metabolism
3. Boosts your energy
4. Supports sound sleep
5. Helps to keep you from gaining an unhealthy amount of excess weight—which is something that is a concern during pregnancy

Throughout my pregnancy, I did my best to maintain a workout schedule. During the first trimester, I had days of extreme tiredness and an upset stomach—which is normal due to hormonal changes—so I gave myself some grace on those days and didn't work out or just did my stretching workout. But in my second trimester, I kept a regular workout schedule. This included both weight-bearing exercises for strength, toning and metabolism-boosting, and aerobic exercises for endurance. In addition, I enjoyed my stretching routines to help keep my bones and muscles flexible and help prevent injury.[1]

A MOTHER'S PRAYER FOR WEEK 21

Dear Lord, I pray for my baby's bones that are developing this week so they can produce life-giving blood cells. I ask You for bone marrow that is 100 percent healthy. I ask for the correct amount of red and white blood cells and platelets.

Lord, You promised to hear and answer our prayers. I claim the promise in Psalm 105:8 that says, "He forever remembers His covenant, the promise He ordained for a thousand generations." You don't forget Your promises, and I thank You for that. You can do all things. You are the Creator of life. My hope is not dependent on myself or other people; You are my Source of strength.

Lord, please give me the strength to eat healthy and to workout. I know that anything I do will benefit my unborn baby. Everything I eat, drink and breathe goes into my baby, so please bless me with endurance and the strength to make the best choices.

And, Lord, I pray that my baby will be happy. Give him or her a heart filled with the joy of being alive. May my child find gladness in everyday things like the sun, a puppy, a kitten, a book and a friend. Give us many happy times together.

In Jesus' name I pray. Amen.

Scriptures for Thought and Meditation

I will sing to the LORD all my life; I will sing praise to my God while I live. May my meditation be pleasing to Him; I will rejoice in the LORD.
PSALM 104:33-34

My soul, praise the LORD, and all that is within me, praise His holy name. My soul, praise the LORD, and do not forget all His benefits.
PSALM 103:1-2

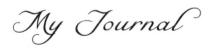

My workout routine before I was pregnant:

_____

_____

_____

_____

_____

_____

_____

_____

_____

_____

My workout routine and energy level now:

_____

_____

_____

_____

_____

_____

_____

_____

_____

What physical issues (weight-bearing exercise, diet, balanced nutrients, rest) I need to work on, and what my game plan is:

_____

_____

_____

_____

_____

_____

_____

_____

Note

1. If you'd like more information about this topic, please see my website, www.PrayFor YourBaby.com.

22

Your Baby Has Favorite Flavors

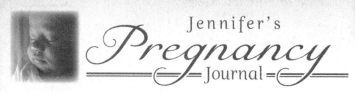

Jennifer's *Pregnancy* Journal

Next week I get to go home to Hawaii to see my mom. I'm so excited! I know it's special for her to see me pregnant, and she has so much wisdom to share. It will be a long flight from Denver, so I'm planning with extra care.

Recently, I read about a plane that was stuck on the tarmac for 12 hours before taking off. How awful for those people! I'll pack an extra bottle of water and snacks, just in case, but I pray that everything will go smoothly on my journey home.

Your Baby's Development

Good things are happening this week. Due to maturing brain cells and nerve endings, your baby's sense of touch becomes more sensitive. The first area to experience more sensitivity is in the cheek, which may explain why your baby starts sucking his or her thumb in the womb. Ultrasound has discovered babies stroking their faces and feeling other parts of their bodies, too, already exploring how they are made. By week 32, nearly every part of baby's body perceives warmth, cold, pressure and pain.

Also this week, your baby gets taste buds. You might wonder if that really means anything now, before your son or daughter is born. The answer is, yes it does. The amniotic fluid surrounding your baby picks up flavors from your food; especially pungent flavors like curry, cumin, garlic, onion and other spicy foods. Research tells us that unborn babies swallow more in response to sweet tastes and swallow less in response to bitter and sour tastes. If you love garlic or hot sauce, perhaps it is because your mother ate spicy food when she was pregnant with you.

During the last trimester, babies swallow up to a liter a day of amniotic fluid, and scientists believe this may serve as a "flavor bridge" to consuming mother's milk, which is also influenced by flavors from the food the mother eats. God set it up so your baby will automatically like the taste of your breast milk.

Babies have a definite sense of taste at birth. Newborns demonstrate having opinions and preferences. Even preemies suck more enthusiastically on a sweetened nipple than on a plain rubber one.[1]

Praying for Your Baby's Happiness

The Bible uses a metaphor of taste to tell us how to be happy. Psalm 34:8 says, "Taste and see that the LORD is good. How happy is the man who takes refuge in Him!" This is a word picture inviting people to the Lord in order to experience happiness. It's interesting that the writer didn't say, "Taste and see if you like it." Instead, he said taste to see, or taste to discover that the Lord is good. In other words, everyone who tries the Lord finds that He is good! A life with God is a life with happiness, because GOD is GOOD.

It's odd now when I look back at the time before I was living for Jesus. I thought I was happy, but in reality, I was just going along on my own, and so much was missing that I didn't even know about. The awesome thing about being a Christian is that we have Jesus as our best friend. We're never alone.

God is so good, and I think that I completely realized this during the first year with our son, Micah. I have never been happier in my life than right now, with my children.

This week, let's pray for your baby's future happiness.

A Mother's Prayer for Week 22

Dear Lord,

Thank You for this week. The time is getting near and I will soon get to see my newborn baby. I am so excited. Lord, help me to read Your Word to my baby, for I know that it is like honey in his mouth. I pray for health and happiness for my child. There is no greater joy for a mother than to see her children walking in the way of the Lord, as it says in 3 John 4.

Give my child true happiness, not through wealth and riches, but from knowing You as his personal Savior. Help me teach my child to read and memorize Your Word and to have a hunger for the Word of Life.

Thank You, Lord, for this beautiful baby growing inside of me. In Jesus' name. Amen.

Scriptures for Thought and Meditation

Like newborn infants, desire the unadulterated spiritual milk, so that you may grow by it in your salvation, since you have tasted that the Lord is good.
1 PETER 2:2-3

How sweet Your word is to my taste—sweeter than honey to my mouth. I gain understanding from Your precepts.
PSALM 119:103

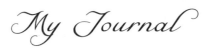

Special flavors and foods I crave during my pregnancy:

_____

_____

_____

_____

What I eat now that I would never have eaten before I was pregnant:

_____

_____

_____

_____

_____

_____

Matthew 5:6: "Blessed are those who hunger and thirst for righteousness, for they will be filled" (*NIV*). What this means to me:

_____

_____

_____

_____

_____

_____

If I plan to travel by air any time during my pregnancy, I need to plan ahead to maximize my comfort and health. In addition to getting up at least every hour to walk around the cabin (for good blood circulation in my extremities), here is my plan and the items I will pack in my travel kit:

- Healthy snacks for a long flight, such as carrots, cucumber slices, celery sticks, dry roasted almonds, cashews and chicken wraps. Put in a small, soft cooler with an ice pack.
- Wear loose, comfortable clothing and easy-to-slip-off-and-on shoes.
- Bring a good book and personal journal for writing.
- Possibly bring an iPod to make the time pass peacefully.
- Bring an extra bottle of water.
- Other items in my travel kit:

Note

1. "Baby's Development of Senses," by Karin A. Bilich, *American Baby*. http://health.discovery.com/centers/pregnancy/americanbaby/senses.html.

Your Baby Prepares to Breathe

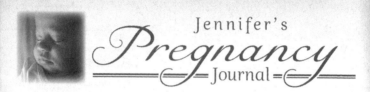

Jennifer's *Pregnancy* Journal

I take a deep breath. This is the best I've felt since the day I got pregnant. Being back home in Hawaii is great! I don't care where you're from, going home again is always something special. Here on the Big Island, the weather is so beautiful—sunny skies and warm temperatures—that I really don't want to go back to Denver, ever.

We're having a fabulous time visiting with my family and enjoying nature—hiking the trails around Waimea, swimming in warm Pacific water, kayaking Kealakekua Bay, and I even rode a boogie board on the tiny waves at Kua Bay. We saw giant sea turtles sunning themselves on the lava rock just south of Kona at Kukio Beach.

Eating a healthy diet is so easy here, because Hawaii has the best sun-ripened fruit—like mangoes, guava, passion fruit or lilikoi, avocados and pineapple—plus, the fresh-caught fish, like ahi (tuna) and mahi mahi.

I feel like I'm back where I belong. Every morning I step outside and take a long, deep breath of the fragrant, tropical air. Paradise!

Your baby's lungs are making huge progress this week, with blood vessels expanding and preparing your child to breathe after birth. Your baby makes breathing movements now, but he or she is just practicing. You still provide oxygen for your son or daughter through the placenta and umbilical cord. A baby's lungs are completely collapsed before birth, but the baby's first breath inflates the lungs and opens up the small air sacs called alveoli, which transfer oxygen to the blood.

Biologists are intrigued by the question, What makes a baby start to breathe on its own? They're thinking that it's a combination of physical stimuli including cold, touch, temperature and oxygen supply; the absence of a protein in the uterus that prohibits breathing; and the baby's own lung maturation. Study is ongoing. I like to think that an angel whispers in the baby's ear and tells him or her it's time to breathe. But either way, it's a wonderful miracle.

Your baby's lungs might also provide a clue as to when you go into labor. A study conducted at UT Southwestern Medical Center in Dallas found evidence that a protein in the unborn baby's lungs could signal it's time to start the birth process.

Although some babies can be born at week 23 and survive, it's better to give more time for lung development and for the other major organs to mature as well. Even so, this week is a milestone.

When Micah was born, the umbilical cord was wrapped around his neck—twice. The doctors think he aspirated, which may have caused "streaking" in his lungs. For two long weeks, I carried him and his little oxygen tank around the house. I had him in a little Moses basket in one hand and the tank in the other. Nurses came to check on him almost every other day, and they all said that he just needed a little help to breathe—something that was not uncommon here in Denver, the Mile High City, with 17 percent less oxygen in its thin air.

I sat and prayed over him every day, that God would make his lungs stronger, and that he would not need the oxygen tank anymore. I claimed the promise in Psalm 34:17: "The righteous cry out, and the LORD hears, and delivers them from all their troubles."

Finally, we went to his two-week checkup, and the doctor said, "Why is he on this? He's perfectly fine."

God answered our prayers! We were ecstatic!

Ten days later, when he was three-and-a-half weeks old, Micah and I boarded a plane and flew to Hawaii to visit my parents. They had such a wonderful time meeting their new grandson.

God is our oxygen. He is our Breath of Life. Without Him, we cannot live. Genesis 2:7 tells us that God formed man and breathed into his nostrils, and the man became a living being. That is amazing to me.

When your new one enters this world, you wait to hear your baby's cry. Every mother does, waiting to hear the sound of her child's voice for confirmation that breath and life has occurred. Malia had no problem with that. She screamed like bloody murder! And she still does when she doesn't get her way. She definitely has a strong will and a strong set of lungs!

A MOTHER'S PRAYER FOR WEEK 23

Dear Lord,

I thank You for breathing the breath of life into my baby. You are amazing, God, and I acknowledge Your greatness and praise You.

Lord, please help my baby's lungs to continue to grow and develop and to form perfectly. Help me carry the baby to full term so the lungs and other organs have time to mature. Give my baby strong and healthy lungs, and strength and health in every way.

Lord, let us all use the breath You have given us to express gratitude and praise to You. And let us use the breath You've given us to pass on Your love to others. Help me to be a good role model for my family, and help me to be an expression of Your Holy Spirit. Thank You, Lord.

In Jesus' name I pray. Amen.

Scriptures for Thought and Meditation

Then the LORD God formed the man out of the dust from the ground and breathed the breath of life into his nostrils, and the man became a living being.
GENESIS 2:7

Hallelujah! Sing to the LORD a new song, His praise in the assembly of the godly. Let Israel celebrate its Maker; let the children of Zion rejoice in their

King. Let them praise His name with dancing and make music to Him with tambourine and lyre. For the LORD takes pleasure in His people; He adorns the humble with salvation. Let the godly celebrate in triumphal glory; let them shout for joy on their beds. Let the exaltation of God be in their mouths.
PSALM 149:1-6

My Journal

This week, as I think about my baby's lungs developing to be able to breathe after birth, here is what I found out about the Holy Spirit's work in me, so that I can "breathe" in a spiritually hostile environment.

What the indwelling Holy Spirit moves me to do (read Ezekiel 36:27):

_____

_____

_____

What helps my spiritual lungs mature (read Romans 8:9-18):

_____

_____

_____

The reason I follow God's laws for a healthy body, mind and spirit (read 1 Corinthians 6:19-20):

_____

_____

_____

The finishing touch to the book of Psalms is, "Let everything that breathes praise the LORD. Hallelujah!" (150:6). I can be a role model and teach my child to praise the Lord by:

_____

_____

_____

Your Baby's Balance

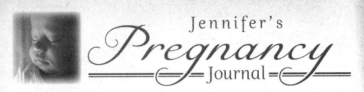

Jennifer's *Pregnancy* Journal

All good things must come to an end. We're back in Colorado, and I have to face the reality of not living in 80-degree weather year round. We hope to move there one day and run our nonprofit organization, Agape Ranch (www.AgapeRanchHawaii.org), a haven for cancer patients. Our goal is to bring people from around the globe to a ranch in Hawaii for a week of learning, support, relaxation and healing. When it's built, our plan is for Dan and me to teach nutrition and exercise classes, and to have experts come and share their knowledge: everything from new medical innovations to fighting cancer with alternative approaches utilizing proper eating and exercise to strengthen the immune system. But, most important, we want to introduce them to Jesus Christ.

That's one of our long-term dreams—to spread joy by giving generously to others. But my dream right now is my baby!

Scientists who study otolaryngology (the medical specialty concerned with ear, nose and throat) tell us the basic structure of the inner ear is present in unborn babies at 24 weeks. This means your baby can now hear and detect direction of motion, such as turning forward to backward, side to side, and up and down.

At this point, there's still enough room for baby to turn upside down and back again—and he can tell which way is which. Some people have an extraordinary sense of direction, and they rarely get lost. You may know someone like that.

Because the inner ear is located close to the center of the skull, it is one of the best-protected sensory systems we have. It seems that God made it a priority to safeguard our hearing and balance. One of the things I want for my children is to have a good sense of balance when it comes to life management.

In my area of fitness, I see people who go overboard, one way or the other. There are the people who never exercise beyond walking from the bedroom to the refrigerator. They totally neglect their bodies. On the other extreme, there are people who make getting in tip-top shape their number one priority in life, and they neglect other important things like studying God's Word, spending time in prayer and worshiping God with other believers. I was one of those people before I was following Christ.

In other areas, too, people get out of balance. We all know workaholics and people who are too lazy to go to work at all. Any type of obsession is out-of-balance behavior, and eventually will cause harm.

I believe that part of living a balanced life includes thinking beyond ourselves and giving to others.

A Heart of Generosity

There is no greater joy than giving to others, so I also want my children to learn about generosity at an early age. My grandma is one of the most generous people I know. When I was young, she brought us suitcases of gifts from Chicago, all the way to Hawaii. Anything we asked for she would find and tuck away until her next trip. She barely brought anything in her bags for herself—it was always about us. And fortunately for us, she was able to visit three or four times a year, because her son worked for United Airlines, and she got to fly for free for many years.

Grandma treated each of her grandchildren the same, showering them with love by giving, and she did the same for her "adopted" grandchildren and others she met along life's way. She also gave to charities; and even later, when money was short for her, she never stopped giving to charities or to us kids. Through her generosity,

Grandma made a lasting impression on me, and I want to be this kind of role model so my children will grow up to be giving people.

A MOTHER'S PRAYER FOR WEEK 24

Dear Lord,

It's amazing how You think of everything. You've placed each part where it should be. I pray for good hearing and a good sense of direction for my baby. Please keep my baby's ears safe and help him not to get earaches, as many young children do.

Lord, please give my baby a good sense of balance in life. Let him know what is important and yet not go overboard or be obsessive. Give him the wisdom to know when to work, when to rest and when to play. Let him know that with a balanced Christian life, following Your ways, there is a time for everything.

Thank You, Lord, for this gift of life. Please also help me to balance my own life according to Your will. Help me to know when to rest and just leave the undone housework alone. Help me to know when to say no to requests from other people. Help me take time to pray and meditate on Your Word. Let me be a good role model of living a balanced Christian life.

And, Jesus, please help me teach my children to be generous. It's hard sometimes in this society we live in, but You showed us examples all throughout the Bible on how we should give to others. Help me to be a good example.

In Messiah's name. Amen.

Scripture for Thought and Meditation

Good will come to him who is generous and lends freely.
PSALM 112:5, *NIV*

A generous man will prosper; he who refreshes others will himself be refreshed.
PROVERBS 11:25, *NIV*

My Journal

I do a good job of balancing these areas of my life:

_____

_____

_____

_____

_____

_____

I need to work on finding balance in the following areas:

_____

_____

_____

_____

_____

_____

I show generosity to others by:

_____

_____

_____

_____

_____

_____

I will show generosity of my time and resources to my child by giving up:

_____

_____

_____

_____

_____

_____

_____

25

One-of-a-Kind Fingerprints

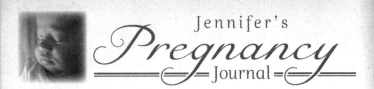

Jennifer's *Pregnancy* Journal

A big snowfall blew in, so we made the best of it and went sledding. I was very careful and just went down the little hills, but I'm sure the baby liked it—he was kicking up a storm!

Another significant event of the week was finding our doula.[1] Her name is Janet, and she is also from Hawaii. She will be helping me before, during and after the birth. We really clicked, so I think I'm going to like having her help me during this very special time. I know that God has placed her in my life for a reason. Not sure what the reason is yet, but this is a God-thing. I just know it.

Another person who has been a tremendous help to me is my dear friend Betty, my massage therapist. Her daughter went to school with my little brother. She is a mother of three herself, and during my massage sessions, she gives me a pep talk about how beautiful I am pregnant and how great a mom I'm going to be. She has been a godsend, helping me get through this time with a positive attitude.

Your baby's hands are now fully formed: 10 exquisite fingers, complete with miniature fingernails and even fingerprints. The pattern of loops, whorls and arches your baby has on her fingers are her permanent, unique pattern. Not even identical twins have the same fingerprints. Identical twins have the same DNA, but not the same fingerprints.

Interestingly, about 1,750 years before the birth of Christ, Babylonians used fingerprints to sign their clay tablets; so even then, they knew people had individual patterns to the ridges on their fingers.

For me, the fingers and hands are one of the most important parts of my baby's body. You'll remember that Helen Keller, a brilliant woman who was born blind, deaf and mute, learned to read, "hear" and "speak" by using the tips of her fingers in the palm of another person's hand, and vice versa.

One of my favorite memories of Micah when he was just a little love bug is when he'd come and pet my face with his sticky little hands. He touched my cheeks and hair and said, "I love you, Mama." My heart just melted every time. I'd think, *I don't deserve such a wonderful little boy.* But when I was still pregnant with him, I prayed diligently that he would always use his hands to help others and never use them for hurting anyone. And now that he has a little sister, I can see that God heard my prayers. To this day, Micah has never hit or hurt Malia. He'll walk up to her, touch her cheeks and give her a kiss. I believe he will use his hands to protect her when they get older and that he will never harm her. So I encourage you, too, to pray for how your baby will use his or her hands.

If your baby already has a brother or sister or may have one in the future, it's good to pray for their relationship. As a parent, you have the authority to stand for your children in prayer. Take hold of faith and proclaim peace and joy in your household, in Jesus' name.

A MOTHER'S PRAYER FOR WEEK 25

Dear Lord,

Thank You for creating each of us as unique individuals, including our own unique fingerprints. I pray for my baby's hands and fingers. Lord, help him to use his hands only for good and never for harm. Help him to be kind and gentle. Help him to use whatever talents You may give him, whether it's music, writing, sports or whatever, to be a blessing to others and to You.

As it says in the psalms, may my baby praise You with his hands by lifting them to You during times of worship. And, Lord, I claim Deuteronomy 2:7 that says, "The LORD your God has blessed you in all the work of your hands."

Lord, I also pray for the siblings. Help all of the children to get along with one another and grow up to be close friends. I pray they will look out for each other and use their hands only for good.
In Jesus' name. Amen.

Scriptures for Thought and Meditation

Your hands made me and formed me; give me understanding so that I can learn Your commands.
PSALM 119:73

The Lord your God has blessed you in all the work of your hands.
DEUTERONOMY 2:7

My Journal

Fingerprints are one of the ways a person is unique. Some unique qualities in our family that my baby may inherit are:

_____

_____

_____

_____

_____

_____

My Fingerprints (use ink from a stamp pad or watercolor finger paint to put your fingerprints here):

```
┌─────────────────────────────────────────┐
│                                          │
│                                          │
│                                          │
│                                          │
└─────────────────────────────────────────┘
```

Note

1. A doula is a professional trained in childbirth who provides emotional, physical and informational support to the woman who is expecting. The doula's role is to help women have a safe, memorable and empowering birthing experience.

26

Your Baby Sees

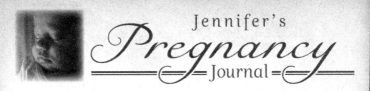

Jennifer's **Pregnancy** *Journal*

Daddy Dan is nesting this week! I thought I'd be the one to nest, but it's definitely him. He has finished the entire basement and put in a large gym where we can train our clients; he has added an office/guest room and installed a full bathroom. The entire remodel took less than three weeks to complete because Dan acted as the foreman and called the guys every day to make sure they showed up and worked.

As if that wasn't enough, now he's talking about ripping out the carpet in the living room and bedrooms, replacing it and then installing hardwood floors in the entire upstairs. It's sweet of him, because he wants to do it for my benefit. He says it will help eliminate the bad allergic reactions I have to dust and molds and will keep our house a lot cleaner. I'm sure he's right, but the thought of a construction crew working in the house right now is not appealing, though it would be nice to have it done.

Can your baby see inside your womb?

Yes! At about week 26 to 28, depending on your individual baby's growth, your baby will open his or her eyes and see for the very first time.

Vision is the last sense to mature. Up until now, a baby's eyes are sealed shut while the retinas develop; but during weeks 26 to 28, your baby will open his or her eyes. Babies even blink their eyelids.

What's more, doctors have detected as early as week 26 that a set of twins will open their eyes, blink, look at one another, reach out and touch one another's faces—and then hold hands. How sweet is that!

Remember the Old Testament account of the twins Esau and Jacob being born (see Genesis 25)? As you may recall, Rebekah could not conceive; so her husband, Isaac, prayed to the Lord on her behalf, and she became pregnant—an excellent example of intercessory prayer. Back then, there were no ultrasound machines to detect twins, so when Rebekah felt some strange action going on, she went to the Lord and inquired, "Why is this happening to me?"

And the Lord basically said, "You have twins who are engaging in sibling rivalry. Your two sons will grow up to become the fathers of two nations."

As they were born, the second son, Jacob, came out holding on to his brother Esau's heel, as if to say, "Hey, I've got you, and I'm ready to compete with you." Undoubtedly, Rebekah's twins could see one another before they were born.

Just as it's not totally silent inside your womb, neither is it totally dark. A small amount of light filters through if you're out in the sun or under bright lights. However, you should never shine a bright light, such as a flashlight, into your abdomen, because light that strong can permanently damage the part of your baby's brain that interprets sight. But the point is, medical science has confirmed that babies can see during this time in your pregnancy, and I think that's fantastic.

I prayed for my baby's eyesight this week, but I took it a step further and prayed for his spiritual sight as well. We see or perceive God, not with our physical eyes but with "the eyes of our heart." That's a beautiful metaphor that comes from Ephesians 1:18-19 where the apostle Paul wrote, "I pray that the eyes of your heart may be enlightened so you may know what is the hope of His calling, what are the glorious riches of His inheritance among the saints, and what is the immeasurable greatness of His power to us who believe, according to the working of His vast strength." Use powerful Scripture this week as your model for praying for your baby's spiritual sight.

A MOTHER'S PRAYER FOR WEEK 26

Father God,

I thank You for giving us spiritual insight through Your Word. I pray that my baby will grow to have sharp spiritual vision.

May he experience Your calling on his life at an early age. Open the eyes of his heart and enlighten his mind with Your Word. Fill his life with the glorious riches that are the inheritance of Your people. Fill his life with love, joy, peace, patience, kindness, goodness and temperance. As his mother, I stand for him in prayer and claim the promises in the Bible for him.

And, Lord, I pray for my baby's eyes that they will open and see this week or sometime very soon, according to what is right for his development. Please give my child perfect vision. If there is anything that threatens my baby's sight, I ask You to heal him right now and create a perfect retina, optical nerve and perfect interpretation of the image displayed in his brain.

And, Lord, I pray that if I'm having twins, they will have a special relationship and become close friends right from the beginning. Give them a bond that cannot be broken.

In Jesus' name. Amen.

Scriptures for Thought and Meditation

Bright eyes cheer the heart; good news strengthens the bones.
PROVERBS 15:30

I pray that the eyes of your heart may be enlightened so you may know what is the hope of His calling, what are the glorious riches of His inheritance among the saints.
EPHESIANS 1:18

My Journal

What the metaphor "open the eyes of my heart" means to me:

_____

_____

_____

_____

_____

_____

_____

_____

_____

_____

_____

_____

_____

If there was a special time when God opened your spiritual vision, journal that now so that you can read it with your child when he/she is old enough to understand.

_____

_____

_____

_____

_____

_____

_____

_____

_____

_____

_____

_____

_____

27

Resting in God

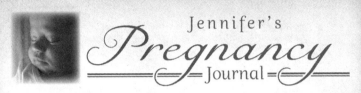

Jennifer's
Pregnancy
Journal

This is the best week of my pregnancy so far. We are back in Hawaii visiting my mom and dad and the rest of the family.

We're staying at our favorite hotel again, The Hilton Waikoloa on the Big Island. They have great pools with water slides, a kids' beach and a dolphin pond. This is where Dan and I got married, and we try to come back every year if possible.

We've been swimming every day, and Micah is learning fast. He's like a little fish or, according to him, a shark. Still, I put the water wings on him just in case. He's only two, and he thinks he can swim, but then all of a sudden he'll go under, so I'd rather be safe than sorry.

The best thing about being on vacation is that I sleep better here. I'm not sure if it's the stress-free attitude that comes along with not having to be concerned about anything except where our next meal is going to be or what pool to enjoy today—but it's sure been relaxing.

As your pregnancy progresses, it may become more difficult to get a good night's rest. There are multiple reasons you may have trouble sleeping at some point in the nine months of your pregnancy. Here are 15 common sleep stealers:

1. Can't get comfortable
2. Exercise before bed keys you up
3. Frequent urination

4. Heartburn and indigestion
5. Hunger
6. Insomnia
7. Leg cramps
8. Medications
9. Nausea
10. Restless legs syndrome
11. Sharing a bed
12. Sleep apnea
13. Snoring and congestion
14. Vivid dreams
15. Worrying about your baby

I experienced 13 of the 15 listed here. The funniest one was the restless legs syndrome. One night, my husband woke me up and said I was kicking him; but of course, I didn't remember anything. The next night, I woke up with three big pillows in between us. I guess he was serious!

I love what Jesus said about being worn out in: "Come to Me, all of you who are weary and burdened, and I will give you rest" (Matthew 11:28).

Psalm 4:8 says, "I will both lie down and sleep in peace, for You alone, LORD, make me live in safety."

Any anxiety we have we can give to God. Any worries we have about our baby's sleep we can just ask God to give us peace about.

After Micah was born, the first question I remember people asking was if my baby was sleeping through the night. Since he was my first baby, I never thought of praying for his sleep while I was pregnant. Well then, it seemed that he practically never slept. He woke up almost every hour to nurse, for the entire first year. It seemed that I had no choice but to keep him in my bed.

I didn't make the same mistake twice. With Malia, I prayed and prayed for a good sleep pattern right from the beginning. And wouldn't you know it, God answered my prayer right away. The first week, she pretty much slept the whole time, which is normal; but by the second week, she gave me six to eight hours of sleep a night. It was wonderful! But once she started teething . . . well, that's another story.

Sleep, or lack of it, affects your ability to function, and it affects your baby's growth. This week ask for God's grace and for restful sleep for you and your baby.

A MOTHER'S PRAYER FOR WEEK 27

Dear Lord,

You gave us sleep as a time for rest and renewal. You showed us by example when You created the world and took the seventh day to rest. Lord, please help me, tonight and from this time forward, to get a deep and rejuvenating sleep. If I wake up in the middle of the night, please help me to go right back to sleep.

Lord, please help my baby to develop good sleep patterns from the very beginning. I pray for safety while my baby sleeps. Protect her from SIDS or any other harm. Let your angels watch over her all through the night—and the daytime too.

Bless my baby whether in her crib or by my side, or in the car seat. Anywhere she sleeps, make it relaxing and peaceful.

Lord, You promise us in Isaiah 26:3 to keep our minds in perfect peace when we trust in You. Help me keep my focus and trust in You and cast out all fears. I choose peace of mind. I choose to trust in You, Lord Jesus, because I know You love me and my baby with an ever-lasting love. I receive Your peace right now. Thank You, Jesus. Amen.

Scriptures for Thought and Meditation

For he grants sleep to those he loves.
PSALM 127:2, *NIV*

You will keep him in perfect peace, whose mind is stayed on You, because he trusts in You.
ISAIAH 26:3, *NKJV*

My Journal

Things I worry about that keep me awake:

_____

_____

_____

_____

_____

_____

Based on any of these Scripture passages (Psalm 23; Proverbs 3:5-8; Matthew 6:25-27; Philippians 4:6-7; 1 Peter 5:7-11), I have concluded that the antidote to worry is:

_____

_____

_____

_____

_____

I can make some choices for my body, mind and emotions that will encourage a good night's rest (listening to soothing instrumental music before bed, reading a comforting passage from God's Word, eating a protein snack before bed instead of something sugary or containing caffeine). Here's what I will do the next time I can't sleep:

_____

_____

_____

_____

_____

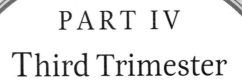

PART IV

Third Trimester

WEEK 28 TO BIRTH

All the days ordained for me
were written in your book
before one of them came to be.
PSALM 139:16, NIV

28

Creating Your Birth Plan

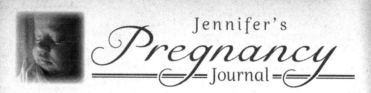

Jennifer's *Pregnancy* Journal

I was able to get outside for walks more this week, and the exercise felt great. Something funny happened too. My friends gave me a jogging stroller for a baby gift, and since I don't have a baby to fill it yet, for added resistance I popped a 15-pound bag of birdseed in the stroller. Then I pushed it up and down the hills around our neighborhood for a great workout. It so happened that a senior couple was out for a stroll, and when they saw me coming up the road with the baby jogger, they got excited. They wanted to stop and peek at the cute baby! When they looked in and saw the bag of birdseed, well, the look on their faces was priceless. They were quite confused until I explained I was still pregnant and out for some exercise. We all had a good laugh!

Another thing we did this week was create my birth plan. My doula Janet, Dan, and I sat outside on the patio and discussed all of our options for the birth. The purpose is to be fully prepared and therefore avoid any misunderstanding later. It feels good to know that I have choices when it comes to my baby's birth.

The third trimester means your baby is almost here! Now it's time to create a birth plan to prepare for your labor and delivery. You may already know how you'd like the birth experience to go, but there are many choices and options to consider.

Birth Story from the International House of Prayer

The house is quiet. Christmas lights sparkle on the tree, and the rain splatters on the window outside. Our baby daughter is napping peacefully in her crib. As I reflect on our journey of waiting for her, I am so grateful to God.

For years, I'd been longing for a child. Disappointed in not becoming pregnant, I wrestled with jealousy as I watched friends announce their pregnancies. I feared that I'd never have a baby of my own. Then, during a flight from Albuquerque to Kansas City, my husband "coincidentally" met two members of the International House of Prayer staff. They invited us to visit the prenatal prayer rooms at IHOP, and we accepted.

On November 9, 2006, we received personal prayer and Holy Communion.

In December, our internship drew to a close. Todd, a dear friend and fellow intern, prophesied over us, "I feel that you are leaving with a child . . ." At the time, I thought this was about some sort of spiritual gift, the new thing that God had "birthed" in our hearts during our time at IHOP. I was not thinking of a literal baby.

And then on December 13, we found out that we were pregnant! It was unreal at first, and then we were ecstatic, amazed and full of joy at God's faithfulness! What fun we had telling our parents and friends!

My birth plan included my preference for natural childbirth, praise and worship music and my friend who is a nurse to come visit. During my labor and delivery, God was right there with me.

My labor lasted 42 hours. That long labor was a surprise, but I didn't want to get uptight about my birth plan, so I decided to go with the flow and trust God. When the doctor suggested I have an epidural, I agreed. When I started feeling discouraged, my Christian nurse friend came and lifted my spirits. Right up until it was time for me to push, we played praise and worship music, which brought the Spirit of the Lord into the room.

Another blessing was that my husband's mother was with us. When our baby was born, she was able to hold our daughter right away and say, "I'm so glad you're finally here! I've been waiting for you all these hours, just so I could greet you when you first came into the world. Welcome, baby." My mother-in-law brought so much joy into the room—it was powerful!

We wanted to give our daughter a name with a special meaning. We chose Cosette, which means "of the victorious people." She is an incredible joy to us. Through this experience, the Lord taught me to truly trust in Him.[1]

How to Create a Birth Plan

The best plan is to have a plan, so start jotting down ideas now and get your husband and health care provider involved too. Here are some things to consider:

- Where will the birth take place? A hospital, birthing center, or at home?
- What medication will I use, or do I prefer natural childbirth?
- What birthing positions would I like?
- Who will be allowed in the room with me?
- What will I wear?
- Do I want music played? Scriptures read?
- Will I breastfeed my baby?
- If it's a boy, will he be circumcised?

By creating a birth plan, you'll have peace of mind knowing that your preferences are clearly spelled out. Yes, something unexpected may come up, and if that happens, you'll adapt like Holly Montoya did in the story on page 147, and you can even create "what ifs" into your birth plan. (To print out a free, easy-to-use birth plan form, go to www.PrayForYour Baby.com. You can make changes as you work through your ideas, and then when you're finished, print out copies for your practitioner, nurse, doula, husband, and one to keep for your baby book.)

A MOTHER'S PRAYER FOR WEEK 28

Lord Jesus,

Thank You for helping me make it this far in my pregnancy, and for the way You will help me through these final months. Help me increase my prayer time and hear Your Holy Spirit as You speak back to me. Help me recognize Your voice and understand what You say. Continue to teach me to be open to You and to trust in You.

And, Lord, protect me from complications in pregnancy. Safeguard my health and my baby's health. Protect me from unnecessary scares and fear. Lord, Your Word says perfect love casts out fear. I accept Your love and the peace of the Holy Spirit. I put my life in Your hands, and I will not fear.

I pray for my baby's continued growth during this final trimester. Lead and guide me as I prepare my birth plan.

I praise Your holy name, Jesus. Amen.

Scriptures for Thought and Meditation

Don't worry about anything, but in everything, through prayer and petition with thanksgiving, let your requests be made known to God. And the peace of God, which surpasses every thought, will guard your hearts and your minds in Christ Jesus.

PHILIPPIANS 4:6-7

You keep him in perfect peace whose mind is stayed on you, because he trusts in you.

ISAIAH 26:3, ESV

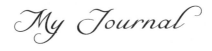

My Journal

How I feel about being in my third trimester:

_____

_____

_____

_____

_____

_____

_____

_____

_____

An answer to prayer I am grateful for:

_____

_____

_____

_____

_____

_____

_____

_____

_____

_____

_____

Print out and insert your birth plan here:

Note

1. This is an excerpt adapted from a pregnancy journal entry from Holly Montoya.

29

Your Baby Hears You!

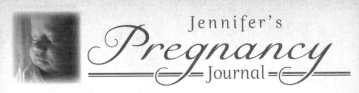

Jennifer's
Pregnancy
Journal

This week was Mother's Day. I got to thinking that this same time next year, I'll be celebrating MY FIRST MOTHER'S DAY! How exciting! My baby will be about 10 months old or so. Great age . . . maybe we'll go to brunch. I can't wait! And they always have something special in church, too, like a video of the moms and kids. Really cute stuff. Soon, I'll get to be a part of it.

Maybe my child will color me a picture when he's old enough. I can't wait to see all the things he's going to do. I'm looking forward to reading him stories. I love a good story, and I'm sure my children will as well.

Newborn babies recognize their mother's voice. It's a fact that's been widely accepted for many years. So let's think about that: How can a baby recognize her mother's voice five seconds after she's born? The logical line of thought is that she must have been able to hear her mother speaking before she was born. True enough, but the science community did not have hard evidence that it was so until an exciting, groundbreaking research project was completed in May 2003.

The study took place in China among 60 pregnant women, and the findings were published in the May issue of *Psychological Sciences* by lead researcher Barbara Kisilevsky, Ph.D., of Queens University in Ontario, Canada, who conducted the study with the Chinese researchers. Since then, it has been reviewed and cited by medical doctors and doctors of science all around the world. So, here's what happened . . .

The mothers read a two-minute poem into a recorder. For half of the unborn babies, they played the voices of their mothers reading the poem; for the other half of the unborn babies, they played the same poem recorded by a woman other than the babies' mothers. The question was, would the babies react differently to the sound of their own mother's voice when the same words were played?

When the tape of a baby's mother's voice was held next to her abdomen, the baby's heart rate increased throughout the entire recording and remained high for the next two minutes as well. But when another woman's voice was played at the same volume, the baby's heart rate decreased and remained lower throughout and after the recording. In both groups, the changes to the babies' heart rates began about 20 seconds into the recording, which shows they were reacting to the recording.

Lead researcher Barbara Kisilevsky, Ph.D., said, "They get excited when they hear their mother's voice; it is something that they recognize and are aroused by. What this study shows is that the babies had to recognize and distinguish between the two voices in order to respond differently."

In an interview with WebMD, she also said, "This is an exciting finding, because it provides evidence of sustained attention, memory and learning by the fetus."

In a different research project, Anthony DeCasper, Ph.D., psychologist at the University of North Carolina, discovered that babies react differently to different stories, even when read by the same mother.

That tells me the babies recognize their own mother's voice, and they distinguish between messages.

I don't know about you, but I think this is a lot of exciting proof—and a big dose of inspiration to pray aloud for our babies and to read the Bible aloud. If you're wondering where to start in reading the Bible, I suggest reading the book of Mark in the New Testament, because it's only 16 chapters, and it is the story of Jesus. And then I recommend reading the psalms, which are beautiful poems and songs inspired by God.

Babies recognizing and responding to their own mother's voice reminds me of when Jesus said His people know His voice and follow Him. That's what I want for my children also—to recognize the voice of Jesus and follow Him.

Have you ever walked by an open door and heard the sound of Christian music, and been drawn to it, like you just had to slow down and listen, or even walk inside? I know I have.

After I graduated from college, some friends and I sailed around the South Pacific. One day, we were in Tonga—the oldest and last remaining Polynesian monarchy, located between Fiji and Samoa—and we happened to walk by a small school. The children were singing old hymns, a cappella. I couldn't believe how beautiful the music was! They harmonized like angels. That was almost 20 years ago, but it made such an impression on me, I still remember it today. When you hear music you love, it's like a super strong magnet that draws you, isn't it? That's the way it is for God's people when they hear His message. So this week, I want you to pray not only for your baby's hearing, but also for your baby to hear the voice of the Lord and to respond to Him.

A Mother's Prayer for Week 29

Dear Lord,

I pray for my baby's hearing that is developing now. Give him or her perfect hearing, with the ears and inner parts of the ear working properly. But, Lord, I also pray that my child will hear and recognize Your voice. Give him spiritual ears to hear what You say to his generation, and to him specifically. I pray that my child will love Your voice and be sensitive to it.

Lord, You say in the book of John that Your people hear You and follow You, and that You give them eternal life. I pray now for my child's salvation, that You would give him a wonderful experience in knowing You are his personal Lord and Savior and that You have prepared eternal life for him.

Lord, I also pray that my words express love and are positive, encouraging, life-giving and Bible-based. I pray that my baby hears only good things coming out of my mouth, and I pray that I will think about what I am going to say before I say it. Help me teach by words and action to speak praise.

Show him the path in which You want him to go and help him to spread the Good News of Jesus Christ wherever he goes.

Thank You, Jesus, for hearing my prayer. I ask this in Your name. Amen.

Scriptures for Thought and Meditation

Your faithful love is as high as the heavens; Your faithfulness reaches to the clouds.
PSALM 57:10

My lips will glorify You because Your faithful love is better than life.
PSALM 63:3

My Journal

This is a good week to write out a special message to your baby and then read it aloud. When your child is older, you can look back and read it again together. It's about creating a beautiful moment for you to share together in the future.

My Dear Special Baby, this is what I want to say to you . . .

_____

_____

_____

_____

_____

_____

_____

_____

_____

_____

30

Your Baby's Skeletal Structure

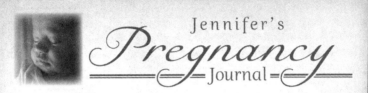

Jennifer's
Pregnancy
Journal

I had a very busy workweek. It's getting harder and harder to hand my clients the weights now that I'm in my third trimester. I actually have them pick up their own weights sometimes if they are too heavy for me. Also, my feet have been sore, especially my right heel, so I'd better get some new shoes soon.

But this was a fun weekend for me. My girlfriends and I went up to the spa at Cordillera in Vail, Colorado. The lodge was inspired by a chateau in Belgium, and it's nestled right below the steep, snow-capped mountains. There are walking trails, indoor and outdoor pools, and the most beautiful pink-orange sunsets at night.

One of my friends has a beautiful home there, so we had a sleepover at her house. I got to swim—something I haven't had an opportunity to do since Hawaii, and it felt great! I wish I had a pool or the ocean nearby—I'd be in it every day!

Swimming is an awesome way for pregnant women to exercise. With the water's buoyancy, you become virtually weightless and cushioned, reducing stress on your joints. Swimming a few laps works all major muscle groups, your heart and your lungs, so I highly recommend it. You can enjoy whatever strokes you feel comfortable with—breaststroke, sidestroke, front crawl or backstroke—as long as you don't strain yourself.

Water jogging or walking is also an awesome workout for your legs and cardiovascular system. It's a good idea to stay about waist deep.

Even if you don't swim, you can participate in water aerobics classes for pregnant women that are offered at many health clubs.

Another advantage of water exercise is that the water helps prevent you from becoming overheated.

Be Safe When You Exercise

When you're pregnant, avoid getting overheated during exercise. Any time that you feel yourself getting too hot, stop and rest. Do not let your heart rate exceed 120 beats per minute. Stop immediately and call your doctor if you start having contractions, and always follow the exercise directions given to you by your doctor or health care provider.

Moms-to-be ask me how hard they can work out during pregnancy. I have a simple answer that can apply to all fitness levels. On a scale of 1 to 10, with 1 being "no challenge" and 10 being "extremely difficult," go for a level of 4 to 5 right now, because you're in your third trimester and don't want to overdo it. The key here is just to get you up and moving on a daily basis. (For more information on fitness tips while you're pregnant, see my website, www.PrayForYourBaby.com.)

Take Time to be Healthy

Some women feel like they're being self-centered when they take time out for themselves to exercise, but that's not true. Your baby also benefits when you exercise. What's more, you need to take care of yourself if you're going to take good care of your child. I try not to feel bad about doing something good for myself, because I know it helps me be a patient mommy and that Micah and Malia will benefit in the end. I know it's not always easy; as I said, I try, but sometimes I don't follow my own advice!

Your Baby Needs Protein, Calcium and Iron

Another way you can help your baby's skeletal structure to grow strong is by getting enough protein, calcium and iron.

It's important to know that your baby relies on you for all his iron, which he stores up to last him for the first six months of life. If you lack iron, your baby will be served first, and then you may suffer from fatigue, headaches and difficulty concentrating. Fortunately, your body absorbs calcium better now than before you were pregnant—thank God for that—especially in this last half of pregnancy, when your baby needs the most calcium and is growing rapidly.

When you take good care of your body, you feel better on the inside as well. If you're like me, it's easier to have patience when you're feeling good. I know it's hard to wait so long for your baby to come. Patience is not my strongest characteristic, so there were times when I had to rely on the Lord to help me. I think of Romans 5:3-4:

> Suffering produces endurance, and endurance produces character, and character produces hope (*ESV*).

When you feel like you're suffering with various discomforts due to pregnancy, realize that you are building endurance and character, and then take comfort in the hope that it will all be worth it when you hold your baby in your arms. I can say this from experience, because my second pregnancy with Malia was very difficult. I had so many challenges, from hernias to sciatica. I've never been through so much pain, but I did my best to praise God through it all—and I can say it was worth it when my daughter was born.

But remember, it takes time and practice to build patience—so don't be impatient! Just keep trusting in the Lord.

A MOTHER'S PRAYER FOR WEEK 30

Dear Lord,
    I praise You for the hard times that stretch my endurance, because I know it's producing good character and working out

patience in me. Help me apply Hebrews 12:1 where it says, "let us run with patience the race that is set before us." I know that applies spiritually, but right now, it also applies to waiting out the time before my baby comes.

I pray that You will help me manifest patience in our home, so that my child will grow up with a good role model. Give my baby a patient spirit, and may he/she be slow to anger and quick to praise.

And, Lord, please continue to help my baby grow strong in every way. And help me take the time to be healthy by exercising.

In Jesus' name. Amen.

Scriptures for Thought and Meditation

But those who trust in the LORD will renew their strength; they will soar on wings like eagles; they will run and not grow weary; they will walk and not faint.
ISAIAH 40:31

For I have learned to be content in whatever circumstances I am.
PHILIPPIANS 4:11

My Journal

I will be good to myself and not feel guilty about it. I will treat myself to:

_____

_____

_____

_____

_____

_____

_____

_____

_____

I can help teach my child to build patience by:

_____

_____

_____

_____

_____

_____

_____

_____

_____

_____

I am patiently waiting on God to tell me this about my child:

_____

_____

_____

_____

_____

_____

_____

_____

_____

_____

_____

_____

_____

_____

31

Your Baby's Immune System

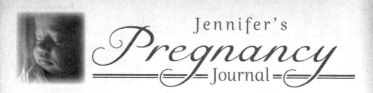

Jennifer's
Pregnancy
Journal

Only nine weeks left and he'll be here! It's getting closer and closer, but the time seems to be creeping by slower and slower.

This week, I spent hours and hours on the baby room. I was up until 3:00 a.m. painting animals on the walls. My girlfriends helped me start the project weeks ago, but I put a lot more time into it than I'd expected. It's looking really cute! I've got a big happy elephant, a mommy and baby giraffe, and two frisky monkeys running down a tree limb. They all match the Zanzibar crib set we have.

I never thought a little baby could consume so much of my thoughts, but I find myself constantly thinking about him and praying for him. I am praying that he will be healthy and have a strong immune system against disease and illness. I'm also praying he will have inner peace and calmness.

By this time, all of your baby's major organs are developed, but the lungs still need to mature in order for your baby to breathe on his own. From here until the birth, your baby will gain weight and strengthen his immune system in preparation for life on the outside.

Your baby's immune system is still not fully mature at birth, but God provided a way for you to help. The antibodies made by your own body's immune system are passed on to your baby when you breastfeed. The La Leche League International is an organization that's been dedicated to the education and support of breastfeeding for more than 50 years. Here is what they say about the benefit of breastfeeding your baby:

> Breastfeeding has been shown to be protective against many illnesses, including painful ear infections, upper and lower respiratory ailment, allergies, intestinal disorders, colds, viruses, staph, strep and e coli infections, diabetes, juvenile rheumatoid arthritis, many childhood cancers, meningitis, pneumonia, urinary tract infections, salmonella, Sudden Infant Death Syndrome as well as lifetime protection from Crohn's Disease, ulcerative colitis, some lymphomas, insulin dependent diabetes, and for girls, breast and ovarian cancer.[1]

I understand that there are valid reasons why some women cannot or choose not to breastfeed their babies; and I am aware that millions of babies who were fed baby formula are strong, healthy and doing very well. So please know that I support the personal decision of all mothers. But my own personal belief is that, ideally, God created mothers to nurse their babies; so I encourage you to consider this option.

I wasn't sure I was going to be able to nurse Micah, but I wanted to try. Then within an hour after he was born, he latched right on and knew what to do. I was so glad, because there is a history of allergies in our family, and breast milk circumvents that problem.

My doctor said nursing helped him to be healthy and quickly gain the weight he needed. Breastfeeding him was a wonderful bonding experience; and now as I write this, I'm nursing Malia, who is just four months old.

Praying for a Calm, Peaceful Baby

In addition to praying for your baby's health and immune system, I also want you to pray that your baby is peaceful and has a calm spirit. We live in a world filled with stress and bad news. Many people live in fear of "what could happen," because they don't know Jesus Christ as their Protector. Yes, bad things happen in the world, but we can stand securely on the promises of God.

First John 4:4 says, "You are from God, little children . . . because the One who is in you is greater than the one who is in the world."

Jesus is called the Prince of Peace (see Isaiah 9:6). Let's pray for our little ones to be calm, peaceful babies and to grow up with an inner peace that comes from above.

Jesus said, "My peace I give to you. I do not give to you as the world gives. Your heart must not be troubled or fearful" (John 14:27).

I'd like to share with you an interesting insight on experiencing peace through silence from Elmer L. Towns, vice president and dean at Liberty University and a Gold Medallion award-winning author. In his book *How to Pray When You Don't Know What to Say*, he writes:

> Do you know that there is power in silence? The power of silence comes not from the absence of words but from the presence of God. When we are silent before God, the Lord can heal us, or build us up, or make us what He intended for us to be: "My soul, wait silently for God alone, for my expectation is from Him" (Ps. 62:5).[2]
>
> We don't have to bang on the door or yell to get God's attention. Too often we think of silence as the absence of noise or just nothing in the room. But silence is something. Silence has its own existence. Just as God exists without being a physical presence, so silence exists for us. When we enter the stillness of our personal sanctuary, we'll find that God is there. He is waiting for us in our silence.[3]

It's usually the mom who sets the mood for the household. When we slow down long enough to enjoy the peace of God, we can share it with others.

A Mother's Prayer for Week 31

Dear Lord Jesus,
Thank You for the privilege of knowing You. Thank You for the peace You give. Lord, I come to You, not frantic or worrying, but with a calm spirit, knowing You are here with me.

I pray that my baby will be born into a peaceful, calm atmosphere and have a peaceful, calm spirit. Help my child to grow up knowing You and having Your peace in her heart, no matter what situations she encounters.

Lord, help me create a secure, calm, peaceful atmosphere in our home—one where love can thrive.

And, dear Lord, I pray that my baby will develop a strong immune system. Protect my child from disease and illness. Help me feed my baby the best way I can; whether it's by breastfeeding or by bottle, help her to get the nourishment she needs on a daily basis.

I praise You and thank You in Jesus' name. Amen.

Scriptures for Thought and Meditation

We have peace with God through our Lord Jesus Christ.
ROMANS 5:1

I wait quietly before God, for my victory comes from him.
PSALM 62:1, *NLT*

My Journal

How I plan to feed my baby:

_____

_____

_____

_____

_____

_____

_____

_____

_____

_____

I can help create peace in our home by taking these concrete actions and creating this kind of atmosphere:

_____

_____

_____

_____

_____

_____

_____

_____

_____

_____

_____

_____

_____

_____

_____

_____

Notes

1. "Can Breastfeeding Prevent Illnesses?" La Leche League International, July 21, 2006.
   www.llli.org/FAQ/prevention.html. For more information about this organization,
   see www.llli.org.
2. Elmer L. Towns, *How to Pray When You Don't Know What to Say* (Ventura, CA: Regal
   Books, 2006), p. 189.
3. Ibid., p. 196.

Baby–Soft Skin

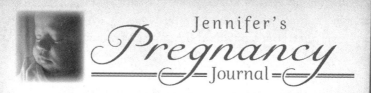

Jennifer's

Pregnancy

Journal

I'm definitely on the home stretch now. Dan tells me I'm doing so well, and he's not sure he would have handled all the physical changes as well as I have; and frankly, I have to agree. But anyway, it feels good to have a husband who appreciates me.

Our house is all torn up now and everything is taped off with plastic to help prevent the dust from spreading during the remodel. It's keeping Dan busy, and I think it helps him cope with the anxiousness of waiting for our baby's birth. This is something he can control. Plus, he wants everything to be nice and in order for the beginning of our new family, and it's something he can be proud of, something that he's done for us.

I've been sleeping downstairs in the new guest room/office because it's nice and cool down there. I had to take our two parrots to the vet to board for the week, as they can't be around the dust or poisonous fumes. We've been airing out the house every night for them, me and for the baby.

I had another appointment with my nurse, and she said I looked great and the baby does too. I'm growing to like her a lot. She's very kind, and she doesn't push me to do any tests I don't agree with.

One thing I wish I could get help with are these spots on my face. They call it the "pregnancy mask"; or doctors refer to it as melasma or choasma. I know it's due to hormones, but it sure looks funny. I hope my baby has flawless skin.

Your baby's skin is looking more beautiful this week. The all-over baby hair is disappearing, and her skin is enviably smooth.

This is a good time to pray that your baby won't develop any of the common newborn baby skin disorders, such as cradle cap or infant acne—even though they aren't serious. God cares for every small detail of our lives, not just the major issues. He knows our thoughts, what we want and need, and He sees everything we go through. Some people fear that God is too busy for "little issues" like temporary rashes, but that's not so. That type of thinking is actually an insult to God, because it puts a limit on His ability to show us compassion and give us good gifts.

God doesn't get "too busy." God is all-powerful and ever-present. He can handle a billion prayer requests at once as easily as He can handle one. God is GOD. He does not experience the limitations of humans; and this means we must not limit our faith in Him or be afraid that our request is too small to "bother" Him with.

If it concerns you, it concerns God, because He loves you.

Think about it this way: If your son or daughter came to you with a burning, itchy rash, would you say, "I'm too busy to think about your pain and suffering"? Or would you say, "That's no big deal; don't bother me with it"? No, of course not. You would stop to look at the rash and do what you could to make it better. The Scriptures say, if you—being a mere human, and a sinner—know how to treat your child right and give him what he needs, don't you think your great and loving God knows how to do the same? Of course! God, who is perfect and is not only loving but *is* also love, will do even better. So never hesitate to ask the Lord for what you and your baby need. Remember, Philippians 4:6 says, "Don't worry about anything, but in everything, through prayer and petition with thanksgiving, let your requests be made known to God."

A Prayer for Joy

In addition to your baby's skin, I'd also like you to pray for your baby to have joy. We don't live in a perfect world; we expect to go through troubles in this life. But that doesn't mean we have to let our joy slip away.

Pray that your child will grow up having a joyful spirit. I love what Nehemiah 8:10 says: "The joy of the LORD is your strength" (*NIV*).

Isn't that fantastic? Our source of strength can be joy! I have to tell you I prayed diligently for Micah to have a spirit of joy; and now everywhere we go, people comment on what a joyful, happy spirit he has. Because their comments are exactly in line with what I prayed for, I take it as an answer to prayer. So be encouraged to pray the same for your baby.

A MOTHER'S PRAYER FOR WEEK 32

Dear Lord,

I pray for my baby's skin. Help it to grow soft and beautiful, the way a baby's skin is supposed to be. And because You said to ask for what we want, I'm asking You to protect my baby from getting any bad skin disorders. Protect her from getting infant acne, cradle cap, jaundice and diaper rashes. Lord, I know those are common skin conditions, but based on Your Word that tells us You care for each and every detail of our lives, I pray that You will protect my baby from those. Give me wisdom and knowledge to do the right things to protect her skin. Help me know which foods and products to avoid so that I can help my child. Help me be a good parent and give her all the care she needs.

But, Lord, even more importantly, I pray that You will fill my child's heart and life with joy. Give her the joy of the Lord and help her to find inner strength as a result of that joy. In all situations, let the joy of the Lord be in her heart. And, Lord, help me to be a role model of joy in my home. Help me bring a spirit of joy into our house.

I love You, Lord, because You are good, and because You are all-powerful and ever-present. Thank You for caring about every detail of my life. I know You are never too busy to hear my prayers, because You are GOD, and You can do all things. You delight in giving good gifts to Your children. You care for us, and I receive that.

In Jesus' name. Amen.

Scriptures for Thought and Meditation

Rejoice in the Lord always. I will say it again: Rejoice! Let your graciousness be known to everyone. The Lord is near. Don't worry about anything, but in everything, through prayer and petition with thanksgiving, let your requests be made known to God. And the peace of God, which surpasses every thought, will guard your hearts and your minds in Christ Jesus.
PHILIPPIANS 4:4-7

I am sure of this, that He who started a good work in you will carry it on to completion until the day of Christ Jesus.
PHILIPPIANS 1:6

Then I will go to the altar of God, to God, my joy and my delight. I will praise you with the harp, O God, my God.
PSALM 43:4, *NIV*

My Journal

I would like my child to find joy in his/her family because:

_____

_____

_____

_____

_____

_____

_____

_____

I would like my child to find joy in his/her early life because:

_____

_____

_____

_____

_____

_____

_____

_____

_____

_____

_____

I would like to find joy in my baby because:

_____

_____

_____

_____

_____

_____

_____

_____

_____

_____

I know God finds joy in me and my baby because:

_____

_____

_____

_____

_____

_____

_____

_____

_____

_____

33

Growing in Faith

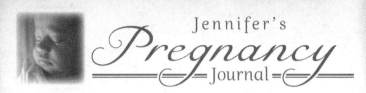

Jennifer's Pregnancy Journal

This weekend I went to another baby shower. It's fun going to my friends' showers, because I'm getting terrific ideas for my shower next week. But this friend is having a girl, just like my other girlfriend, and she got the cutest little pink clothes for baby gifts. I totally loved those baby clothes—but I still want a boy!

Dan signed up for a Daddy Boot Camp. It teaches dads skills like how to change a diaper. I'm sure glad he's going to learn that!

The headline this week for your baby is GROWTH. Not only is she steadily gaining weight, but she's also putting on the fat that's necessary to cope with the climate on the outside; her brain is rapidly growing and maturing as well. Your baby's head will increase by as much as 3/8 of an inch due to brain growth.[1]

Most babies will gain five to nine ounces every week from week 33 until birth.

During this period of tremendous physical growth, it's a good time to focus on growing in faith too. I'd like to share with you a beautiful letter I received from Barb Rickford, of Colorado, while I was writing this book. Here's what she wrote:

"When I still wasn't pregnant at the age of 40, I thought it wasn't going to happen, that it wasn't in God's will. But then while

I was in the process of letting go, I discovered I was pregnant at age 41. Since my journey to become a mom was long and difficult, I've learned the importance and the power of prayer—not only during pregnancy but also before conception and following right through the birth.

"Like Hannah, I prayed for my child, and the Lord granted me what I asked of Him, in His perfect time. So whenever I came across a Bible verse I felt pertained to my child, I prayed it and then wrote the date in my Bible. God promises that His Word, spoken in faith, will not return void, and will accomplish His purpose (see Isaiah 55:11). These are a few of the Scriptures and prayers that guided me in speaking blessing into my child's life—and they still guide me to this day:

Passion: Lord, please instill in my child a soul with a heart for You; a heart that clings passionately to You (Psalm 63:8) and the things that are good, true, noble, lovely, excellent and praiseworthy (see Philippians 4:8).

Purpose: Lord, I pray that my child's life will serve Your purpose in his own generation (see Acts 13:36; Esther 4:14).

Faith: Lord, I pray that faith will find root and grow in my child's heart and that by faith my child may gain what has been promised to him (see Luke 17:5-6; Hebrews 11:1-40). Reveal Yourself to my child at an early age (see 1 Samuel 3:7).

Favor: Lord, I pray that my child will grow in stature and favor with You and with men (see 1 Samuel 2:26).

Courage: Lord, may my child always "be strong and courageous" in his character and actions (see Deuteronomy 31:6).

Contentment: Lord, teach my child "the secret of being content in any and every situation as You give him strength" (see Philippians 4:12-13).

Barb ended her letter by explaining that she believes God's gift of pregnancy wasn't because she deserved this incredible blessing, but that it was God's way of showing His love and His perfect timing. You see, the Rickfords' baby was born on a special day—the exact day of their tenth wedding anniversary.

Barb said, "I've never been filled with such awe and wonder; it was the most euphoric, fulfilling day of my life. Prayer is powerful!"

Thank you, Barb, for sharing your inspiration with all of us. This week, we'll use her letter as inspiration for prayer.

A MOTHER'S PRAYER FOR WEEK 33

Dear Lord, I pray that my baby will find his passion and purpose in life. Lead and guide him right from the start, and reveal Your will to him at an early age. Make Your will clear, and help him never to veer off course from the plan You have for his life.

Help my child obey Your Word and grow in favor with You and with people, so that he might prosper and be blessed.

Give him courage in the face of difficulty. Be his strength and strong tower, as it says in Proverbs 18:10. I pray that my child keeps his focus on You and is fearless, because You are with him.

Grant my child contentment, so that he has a happy heart.

And, Lord, I thank You so much for the blessing of being pregnant with this child. Your Word says every good and perfect gift comes from above. I acknowledge You as the giver of life. I am looking forward to meeting this baby You have given me. I will praise You for as long as I live.

In Jesus' name. Amen.

Scriptures for Thought and Meditation

I will praise You as long as I live;
at Your name, I will lift up my hands.
When, on my bed, I think of You,
I meditate on You during the night watches

because You are my help;
I will rejoice in the shadow of Your wings.
I follow close to You;
Your right hand holds on to me.
PSALM 63:4,6-8

My Journal

The fruit of the Spirit, listed in Galatians 5:22-23, are character qualities Jesus manifested on Earth (He was loving, joyous, peaceful, patient, kind, good, faithful, gentle and self-controlled). Read the Galatians passage and choose a couple of those character qualities to ask God to develop in your child. Here's a simple prayer to begin praying for your unborn baby:

Heavenly Father, I ask that You give my baby the good gifts of being_____ and _____ (choose two of the fruit of the Spirit). May You work those qualities into my child's life, and may my child reflect the character of Christ more and more each day.

What I will do to model these qualities to my child:

_____
_____
_____
_____
_____
_____
_____
_____
_____
_____
_____
_____

In Week 16, I wrote a blessing to speak over my child's pre-birth as well as his or her post-birth. Although I will continue to speak the blessing recorded in Week 16, I have a new blessing to record that better expresses what I want for my child. Here is the new blessing:

_____

_____

_____

_____

_____

_____

_____

_____

_____

_____

_____

_____

_____

_____

_____

_____

Note
1. Women'sHealthCareTopics.com, "33 Weeks Pregnant—Pregnancy Week By Week."

34

Special Gifts

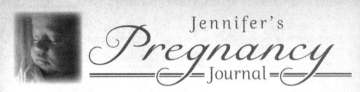

Jennifer's **Pregnancy** Journal

My friend Claire threw me a baby shower Hawaiian style. It was the best ever!! Everything had a tropical theme, from the napkins and plates right down to the slipper mat at the front door. Everyone wore pink and white plumeria leis. Claire created a gorgeous tropical fruit salad and a smorgasbord of other Hawaiian treats. She really went overboard.

I felt so special. I received the most beautiful gifts, even a homemade baby quilt. My parents sent adorable baby outfits for me to open at the shower. Of course I cried. I wish they could have been here.

After it was over, we loaded up my Nissan and—wouldn't you know it—everything wouldn't fit inside. It was hilarious! My neighbor had to transport some of the gifts home for me.

This was an extra special day for me. I feel so blessed that my friends would go to this much thought and effort for me and my baby. This baby is getting more and more real to me, especially looking at the clothes he will wear and the baby gear he'll use. This baby will certainly be loved . . . by a lot of people!

I've been so blessed with the generosity and love of my friends and family that I want to acknowledge them and thank them. I especially want to dedicate this chapter to my brothers and sisters, because without them, life would not be the same. I believe my relationship with my siblings is almost as important as the relationship I have with my parents. As you think about the people in your own life who have been a blessing to you, I'd like to encourage you to take the time to let them know with a hug, a phone call, a greeting card or even an email.

One of the things I like to do to bless someone who has been a blessing to me is give him or her a book. A book is something that's kept and treasured, so it makes a perfect way to say "you're special to me" when you write a personal note inside.

Right from the start, I am trying to teach my children gratitude. I want them to be thankful for every gift, whether it's a birthday present from Grandma and Grandpa or an awesome orange sunset made by God.

Being grateful is a way of living. It's being happy over what you've been given, rather than being discontent about what you don't have.

I like the idea of keeping a Happiness Journal in which you write down something that made you happy that day. For example, your happy moment might be the sighting of a hummingbird, or it could be that you finally got caught up on the laundry. Whatever it is, writing it down is a tangible way of living a life of gratitude and remembering the gifts you've been given.

I know I've mentioned several times how grateful I am for my large family. Please don't feel bad if your own situation is different. If you don't have blood brothers or sisters, you have the Body of Christ. What I mean by that is when you find a church home, God can fill the void by giving you Christian friends. In fact, some people have told me they feel closer to their Christian "sisters" and "brothers" than they do to their natural siblings who don't share their faith. So God has provided a way for us to be a part of His family and to be able to give and receive the support we need. Ephesians 2:19 says that we are "members of God's household." Now that's a wonderful household to be a part of!

I would like to end this chapter by sharing something special from my mother, a woman I love and admire for the way that she tapped into God's strength to raise four boys and three girls. When I asked her if she prayed for us kids when she was pregnant, here is what she wrote:

"I remember praying a lot during each of my pregnancies, but I can't remember all the specifics in regards to what I prayed for each child. (I wish I'd kept a journal.) But I do remember praying for each of you:

Lord, please bless my baby with wisdom and a strong, sound mind. Let him/her be healthy and whole (with 10 fingers and 10 toes, and no abnormalities). Help him/her to grow close to You and trust in You as Savior. Help him/her to become a righteous man/woman who wants to serve You and serve others ahead of himself/herself.

"For some of you, I prayed for your future spouse while you were still in the womb, asking the Lord to bring the special person He had chosen for you into your life at precisely the right time.

"For your brothers and sisters I prayed, 'Heavenly Father, please use my child to spread the gospel around the world to every creature. Help him to always seek first Your kingdom and Your righteousness. Help him to be a witness for You, and give him a desire to do Your will.

"God has answered all these petitions, and many more; He has blessed me and our family far more than I ever envisioned.'"

A MOTHER'S PRAYER FOR WEEK 34

Using my mother's prayer, create your own prayer to God for what you want for your baby. As it was with her, may you look back one day and say, "God has answered all these petitions and many more; He has blessed me and our family far more than I ever envisioned."

Scriptures for Thought and Meditation

So then you are no longer foreigners and strangers, but fellow citizens with the saints, and members of God's household.
EPHESIANS 2:19

Give thanks to the LORD, call on His name;
proclaim His deeds among the peoples.
PSALM 105:1-2

My Journal

I am blessed to be a part of God's family. People I am close to:

_____
_____
_____
_____
_____
_____
_____

As I start a Happiness Journal today, the first three things I want to record in it are:

_____
_____
_____
_____
_____
_____
_____

What makes me happy about carrying my child:

_____
_____
_____
_____
_____
_____
_____

3 5

Time to Prepare for Your Baby's Birth

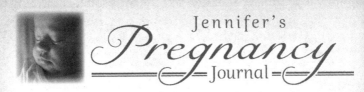

Jennifer's *Pregnancy* Journal

I'm already enjoying the gifts from my baby shower last week. It was so much fun sorting through all the adorable clothes and putting them away in the baby's dresser.

It's been so hot lately, more than 100 degrees. I went and got a great little baby pool to cope with the heat. One of my favorite things to do is sit in the cool water and just relax. So here I am, 35 weeks pregnant, in a swimsuit, in my new little baby pool in the backyard—my poor neighbors! I sure wish I had a picture of that.

This week is Father's Day, and Dan announced he's proceeding with the rest of the remodel plans. What on earth is he thinking? Oh boy!

You're probably thinking a lot about your baby's arrival; hopefully, you're not embarking on a big home project at the same time! But if you are, I can empathize with what you're going through.

This week, your baby weighs about five pounds or more, but he still needs to add fat in order to keep warm enough on the outside. Babies born at this week are usually put in an incubator for added warmth while they grow. Nevertheless, it's getting snug in there, so he doesn't have as much room for doing gymnastics like before. You might notice that he's more active when you're resting, and quieter when you're moving around. This is because you are virtually rocking him to sleep with your movements.

Soon, you'll be rocking him in your arms, so it makes sense to prepare for the delivery at this time.

Get Ready!

This is a good time to make a list so that you won't forget something essential, like your camera, when that big day finally comes. I also recommend packing your bag to take to the hospital or birthing center now, just in case your baby decides to surprise you with an early debut! I like to tell moms-to-be, "Expect the unexpected."

Here's my list of what to take:

- Copies of your birth plan
- A comfortable gown
- Nursing bras and pads
- Nighttime sanitary napkins
- A top to wear when visitors come with their cameras
- Hairbrush, toothbrush, toothpaste and other personal toiletries, including lip moisturizer
- Camera and video camera
- Long-distance calling card or cell phone and phone numbers
- *Praying Through Your Pregnancy* to journal your thoughts (and a pen)
- Your Bible
- Uplifting music (on an iPod)
- Swimsuit for daddy, in case he needs to help you in the shower
- Hair tie
- Water and/or Gatorade or Recharge for you and your support team (After you check in at the hospital, they usually won't let you eat.)
- Stretchy, comfortable clothes to wear home, such as sweat pants and a T-shirt
- Flip-flops or easy slide-in shoes
- Clothes for your baby to wear home
- Baby blankets
- Baby car seat for travel home (required)

And here's one more fun idea:

- Pick up a newspaper on the day of your baby's birth for souvenir headlines and articles[1]

A few comments about clothes to bring: The hospital will provide a gown, but many hospitals will allow you to wear your own, if you prefer. If you live in a cold climate, you might also want warm socks. For your going-home outfit, bring something you fit into when you were about six months pregnant, because it takes a little time for your body to shrink back to its original shape and size. And leave your jewelry at home.

Having your bag packed will be one less last-minute thing you have to do. Other suggestions for getting ready are to have your house in order—*my husband really took that one to heart!*—and to have the laundry done. One mom even suggested getting a good haircut first, because it will be awhile before you can make it into the salon afterward.

This week I want to pray a blessing over you as you make preparations and get ready. Please read this aloud to yourself, from me. Where there is a blank, please fill in your name.

A MOTHER'S PRAYER FOR WEEK 35

Dear Lord Jesus, I thank You for _____ who is reading this book. I thank You for her baby, and that she's made it this far in her pregnancy.

Lord, You know each and every woman who is going to pick up this message and read it. So, I pray that Your Holy Spirit would come right now into the place where _____ is. Let her receive Your Holy Presence right now.

Jesus, I pray that You will bless _____ with joy and gladness as she prepares for her baby's birth. Help her remember what she's learned in her birth classes and what she's read. Help her remember the Scriptures that applied to her. Make Your Word a living testament to _____.

Bless her husband, too, and help him to be the strong support that she needs. If there are other children in the family, bless them with love and gladness.

Help _____ get through these last weeks with a minimal amount of discomfort. Help her sleep through the night in peace. Strengthen her in preparation for the wonderful event of her baby's birth. Give her a quick and manageable delivery, and help this baby to be healthy and perfect in every way. In Jesus' wonderful name I pray. Amen.

Scriptures for Thought and Meditation

Jesus said, "Let the little children come to me, and do not hinder them, for the kingdom of heaven belongs to such as these."
MATTHEW 19:14, *NIV*

Sons are a heritage from the LORD, children a reward from him.
PSALM 127:3, *NIV*

My Journal

My list of things to do before my baby arrives:

_____
_____
_____
_____
_____
_____
_____
_____

Loose-Ends List for the nursery or the house:

_____
_____
_____
_____
_____
_____
_____
_____

Checklist of what I will take to the hospital:

_____

_____

_____

_____

_____

_____

_____

_____

Necessary appointments and arrangements (get that haircut, hire a temporary housekeeper, put pets in a kennel, and so on):

_____

_____

_____

_____

_____

_____

_____

_____

Top 10 names and contact info of people to call/email/text the day of the birth:

_____

_____

_____

_____

_____

_____

_____

Note

1. If you have a great suggestion, please feel free to send me an email. See my website www.PrayForYourBaby.com.

36

Your Baby Gets into Position

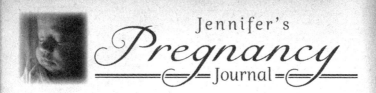

They finished our new hardwood floors, and they're beautiful. Yea!

My husband can be very convincing at times. I never saw people work so hard and so fast. It was just like the remodel of our basement. Dan called the crew every day to make sure they showed up and did what they were supposed to do.

And you know what? I'm so glad we did it.

Once all the dust and fumes were cleared out and I got the place all cleaned up, it looked fantastic. I know it will be a lot healthier for my allergies and for the new baby.

This week was also my thirty-fifth birthday. I can't believe I'm 35. I remember that when I was a teen, the summers never seemed to end. It feels kind of like that with this pregnancy—like it's been forever.

And yet, I have only three weeks to go!!! (Unless the baby comes early!!!!!)

Your baby is getting ready to meet you! By the end of the week, your baby will be considered full term and capable of surviving on his own. Perhaps the most important event for your baby this week is that he stops floating freely and gets into the birth position. Once in position, a baby usually limits his movements to rolling from side to side. However, if your baby happens to be in a bottom down position, or breech, then steps may be taken to try to turn the baby around to avoid having a Cesarean birth.

If you're carrying twins, your babies' birthday could be this week. The National Organization of Mothers of Twins Clubs (NOMOTC) says the average twin birth occurs between 36 and 37 weeks, and the babies weigh an average of five pounds each.

At this point, moms-to-be have one main thing on their mind, which is—you guessed it—my baby is almost here! Because that's pretty much all we're thinking about these days, I want to share with you the inspirational birth stories of a woman named Nancy Rice of Seattle, Washington. Nancy has known my coauthor Carolyn Warren since their college days, and I pray that her story will touch you as it has us.

Nancy's Story

"When I gave birth at home to my daughter Brenda, it was a perfect example of my Christian friends ministering to me." Nancy stopped to laugh at my surprise and then continued, "It was a Body of Christ ministry. It was just really fun!

"Nurse Alice came to guide us through the birth and to be there in case of emergency.

"My friend Amy came, who was the music leader in our church, and she sat at the foot of my bed and prayed—*the entire time I was in labor until Brenda was born—she was there, praying!*

"My friend Laura came, and her role was bringing me words of encouragement that the Lord directed her at just the right times. She seemed to know just what to say, when negative thoughts popped into my mind, to encourage and uplift me.

"I had one other friend there too. Her name was Sheila, and her ministry was running back and forth to bring me popsicles. (Looking back, I should have opted for ice instead; but at the time, it was popsicles.)

"It was really fun!" Nancy laughed with delight at the memory.

"What about your husband? Where was he?"

"He was my breathing coach, and he generally supervised the whole occasion. But there I was, having contractions, and my friends were praying and speaking the Word, and I felt completely surrounded by God's presence.

"God was there with us in the room in such a real way. I felt so taken care of. It was just a wonderful experience going through labor like that.

"And then it came time to push, and there was Amy, still praying—and she literally prayed my baby into this world. Everything went smoothly.

"Our daughter came out peacefully into a room filled with prayers and the sweet presence of the Lord. She didn't cry, she just smacked her lips and looked around. She was peaceful and happy to be here.

"She was delivered by Nurse Alice, Daddy cut the cord and then she was cleaned up. It was like, Brenda is now present and ready to glorify God!

"Now for the rest of the story. Amy, you remember, was the church music leader, and she has since passed on to be with the Lord. Now that Brenda is grown up, she, too, is a worship leader in church and a music teacher. The baton was passed. Isn't that something?"

We think so.

And now here is the story of Nancy's second birth.

The Story of Nancy's Second Baby

"My story of Rhonda's birth is completely different. Two-and-a-half weeks before my due date, I got the strongest nesting urge. I told my husband, Zeak, to go up in the attic and get down the baby clothes.

"He saw no reason to hurry and didn't take immediate action. Normally, I'm pretty calm and laid back, but I absolutely insisted that he go up and get the baby clothes from the attic. He looked surprised, as this was not like me.

"Why are you pushing me?" he asked. He wasn't happy, but he went up and got the clothes, because I wouldn't have it any other way. That evening, he went to bed early, because he was tired. Shortly after, I started labor.

"I didn't want to bother him, because I knew he needed his rest, so I went into Brenda's room—Brenda happened to be spending the night with a friend that day.

"So I was all alone in the room, and my labor and contractions grew stronger and stronger. With each contraction, the Lord's presence came down upon me and lifted me UP. I don't know how else to explain it, but every time I had a contraction, I went up into the Lord's presence, God cushioned each contraction with His Holy Spirit and it was one of the most wonderful, most amazing experiences I've ever had.

"I was still aware that I was having contractions, but it made it so much easier! So it was just me and the Lord, all evening. I would have a contraction and go up into the Lord's presence and feel completely protected by His care for me, and surrounded by His love.

"Finally, I felt close to pushing, so I woke up my husband, and he called the midwife. I got into our waterbed, and while I was waiting for her to arrive, my mouth felt dry—just unbearably dry—so I told Zeak, 'My mouth is dry and I can't do the breathing anymore.'

"Zeak recalled something I'd said previously that I wanted to look presentable, as all women do.

"As I was telling him my mouth was too dry to go on with the breathing exercises, we heard the midwife knock on our door. There was no time to do anything, so Zeak said to me, 'Just smile.' That was his advice—just smile!

"My midwife came into the room, and there I was, sitting on the waterbed, *smiling!*

"She got everything ready as fast as she could, and in 15 minutes, I gave birth to our second beautiful daughter, Rhonda."

Nancy giggled with happiness at the memory and said, "It was both wonderful and funny at the same time!"

Your Birth Story

I wanted to share Nancy's birth stories with you, because it might bring a whole new perspective you hadn't considered before. I know that we read technical and medical information in books and on Internet sites about everything that's happening with our bodies, and we even read about all the things that could possibly go wrong. There's a wealth of information to discover, but I ask you this: When do we read that we can experience God's presence in the delivery room?

When do you hear about bringing your baby into a room filled with the prayers and praises of Jesus? And what about having the Word of God spoken to you as encouragement while you're in labor? I can't help but believe this is the way it should be!

Now please don't misunderstand: I am not advocating home birth over a hospital birth. Both coauthor Carolyn Warren and I delivered our babies in a hospital. But that's not the point. Whether your baby comes at home, in a birthing center, in a hospital or on the operating table via C-section (like Carolyn), the Lord's sweet presence can be right there with you in a real way.

We read in God's Word over and over again that the Lord dwells in the praises of His people. Psalm 22:3 says that the Lord "inhabits" praise. So when we pray and praise Him, His presence comes to us. That's a promise and a spiritual law.

Has it occurred to you that God might come into your delivery room and surround you with His peace and love and make your delivery the most wonderful spiritual experience you've ever had? How awesome would that be!

This week, I want you to pray that our loving Lord and Savior, Jesus Christ, will be right with you, lifting you up into His love during your labor, and that your baby will be born into a room that is filled with His peace and joy. This is my prayer for you. In addition, if you would like me to pray for you by name, please send an email via my website, www.PrayForYourBaby.com.

A Mother's Prayer for Week 36

Dear Lord Jesus, thank You for the privilege of knowing You as our personal Savior and Friend. Thank You for the awesome privilege of praying for the women who read this book. I praise You, because You are a great and wonderful God, full of love and care and understanding for each one of us.

Lord, I pray that You will give the woman reading this book the most wonderful birth experience she ever imagined. Be close to her from the time she goes into labor and throughout. Let her feel You lift her up into Your love during each contraction. Let her know You are with her, helping and guiding her baby to be born. Give her strength and endurance.

And, Jesus, I pray Your holy presence will fill the room as her baby comes into this world. Let there be an atmosphere of joy and gladness, of peace and praise.

Give her an awesome birth experience, one she will treasure forever. In Jesus' name. Amen.

Scriptures for Thought and Meditation

Shout triumphantly to the LORD, all the earth.
Serve the LORD with gladness; come to Him with joyful songs.
Acknowledge that the LORD is God.
He made us, and we are His—His people, the sheep of His pasture.
Enter His gates with thanksgiving and His courts with praise.
Give thanks to Him and praise His name.
For the LORD is good, and His love is eternal;
His faithfulness endures through all generations.
PSALM 100

My Journal

People I can count on to pray for me while I'm in labor (have you asked them to?):

_____

_____

_____

_____

_____

_____

_____

_____

_____

_____

Favorite Scriptures I want to be reminded of while I'm in labor (have you written them out on index cards?):

_____

_____

_____

_____

_____

_____

_____

_____

_____

_____

My thoughts on being close to God during my baby's birth (God will be present!):

_____

_____

_____

_____

_____

_____

_____

_____

_____

_____

_____

37

Put Everything in God's Hands

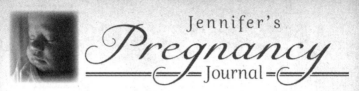

Jennifer's *Pregnancy* Journal

We just got bad news again! I called my doula, Janet, in tears on Thursday, February 28, and left a message to let her know that my baby was breech!

This couldn't be happening. She should have turned already. I didn't want a Cesarean birth. I already went through 30-plus hours of all-natural labor with Micah—no medication. The last thing I wanted now was to go under the surgeon's knife. Why, Lord, is this baby in the breech position? I know You must have a reason; it's just hard for me to understand.

Later, I called Janet back and told her I had another doctor's appointment set for March 6 where they would attempt to do an external cephalic version (a procedure to try to turn a baby from breech to head-down position). So basically, I had one week to turn this baby naturally, or they would do it in the hospital. And then if they were unsuccessful, I would have a C-section birth to prevent possible complications.

I explained all of this to Janet, and she said she'd be happy to go with me, but she also said there are a lot of natural treatments we could try before then.

I prayed: God, I'm so glad You gave me a wonderful Christian woman to help me through this. You are a great God, and I know You have a plan for this baby. Please help this baby turn.

Week 37 was a test of faith for me during my second pregnancy. Actually, the entire pregnancy was more challenging; and because of it, I grew closer to God. Looking back, I know He was in control all along, and I knew I had to just let go and let Him work in a mighty way. Here's what happened.

When I first learned that my baby was in a breech position, it was just two-year-old Micah and me at the doctor's office. Dan was working. I expected nothing more than a simple routine checkup since everything had been fine with the baby for the entire pregnancy. My doctor, who was also pregnant, said how great I was doing, that the baby sounded fine, with a good, strong heartbeat, and that I'd gained just the right amount of weight.

Then she said, "Hey, let's just make sure the head is down."

"Okay, I'm sure it is," I replied. "I've felt hiccups way down there for weeks now."

Micah was standing by my side to see the ultrasound. Then I heard my doctor sigh.

"Oh, no," she said, "your baby is breech. But don't worry—" she continued talking, but I don't think I heard a word she had said after that.

I'm not sure when the tears started flowing. We left the office and got in the car. I called Dan. "Honey, the baby is breech," I said, "and I don't want a C-section!"

I tried to tell him about the procedure to turn the baby that my doctor suggested, but the main thing I remembered was that the procedure itself could cause the water bag to break; and if that occurred, they'd have to perform an emergency C-section.

We called Janet later that evening to let her know what was going on. Then I sent out a mass of emails asking people to please pray for our baby to turn.

Janet came up with a plan of action. Our first order of business would be to try to get the baby to turn on its own. There were options of acupuncture, moxibustion, chiropractic (Webster Technique), lying at an upside-down angle for 10 minutes twice a day, soaking in a warm tub with a bag of frozen peas on top of the abdomen (to entice the baby to turn away from the cold toward the warmth), explaining to the baby that mommy is okay "up here" and needs the baby to turn downwards, and so on.

I thought some of these ideas seemed a bit weird—*but I tried them all!*

All week I prayed; I said God was going to turn this baby one way or the other.

But on Tuesday we went to my appointment, and the baby had still not turned. We saw my doctor, who took into account my feelings and preferences. Right away, she acknowledged she understood that I definitely did not want a Cesarean birth. Whew! That was a relief.

My doctor said she herself had a breech baby with her first pregnancy and had personally had a Cesarean birth. She was now pregnant with her second who was breech and had already scheduled her own repeat Cesarean. I was in awe of how she could so graciously and enthusiastically support me in my wishes to avoid a Cesarean, despite her own rather obvious personal views about the subject. I thought, *What a wonderful doctor!* Please understand that I know there are good, sound reasons for having a C-section birth, and that is a valid choice for some women—it's just that I felt strongly it was not for me.

So then we cleared up questions I had about the cephalic version of turning the baby and scheduled it for two days later on Thursday.

Dan called our pastor, Blake, and he came to our house Wednesday afternoon to pray with us for our baby to turn. Even little Micah participated in the prayer, laying his hand on my tummy, praying for the baby.

I have to admit, I had my doubts at this point. I'd tried everything and was feeling a little discouraged about the situation. So I had to lean on the faith of my family and my pastor. The thing is, we know *Who* holds the future but we don't always know the *whys*. We thought that perhaps the baby *shouldn't* turn, due to a problem with the cord or another possible situation. Or perhaps God was trying to teach me a "life lesson." (Not of my choosing!) Or perhaps there was some other reason we didn't yet understand.

Finally, I had to let go of trying all the various methods of turning the baby, and let go of trying to figure out whether or not she should or shouldn't be turned—*and let God be in control.*

" 'For My thoughts are not your thoughts, and your ways are not My ways.' This is the LORD's declaration" (Isaiah 55:8). I had to trust in God's ways, not my ways.

Thursday, March 6, the day of my doctor's appointment arrived. They were going to try to turn the baby's position.

The nurse set me up on the monitor. Then we waited.

They had two Cesarean deliveries ahead of us that morning. I felt a bit nervous knowing they couldn't just walk in and turn my baby and be done with it. But it wasn't that simple. I had to wait until they were set up to do an emergency C-section on me, just in case it was needed.

I thought, *What if I have my baby today!* I wasn't ready for that. I still had three more weeks to go, and I had things to do.

Then I started thinking and wondering if maybe the baby had turned already. I wasn't sure, but I had felt something funny that morning while I lay in bed. I felt like I was floating in the ocean in Hawaii and a fish swam by, right along my belly. Sort of a swishy feeling. In the meantime, I was starving because I hadn't been allowed to eat since the night before, in case they had to perform the surgery. And now, I wasn't allowed to even sip water. It seemed like the expectation was for the C-section birth.

Would the doctor be successful in turning the baby?

At 10 minutes till noon, the resident doctor walked into our little room and set up the ultrasound machine. As he was talking with me about the procedure, he placed the scanner on my tummy.

Then, just a couple of seconds later, I took a deep breath and the doctor announced, "Your baby's head is down!"

I exclaimed, "Really? Thank You, God!" We were all so excited!

The prayers worked! God was working on our behalf.

"*Hallelujah!* Praise our Almighty God!" We thanked Him and gave Him all the glory. Interestingly, when Pastor Blake prayed for me at home, he had a strong feeling that the baby would turn by the next day, and he was right. I wondered if that was what I felt earlier that morning with the gentle, swishy feeling.

I kept thinking, *Wow, God answered those prayers of faith.* When I was feeling down, my pastor and family stood in for me like a link of faith between God and me. With bolstered faith and praises in our hearts, we went home and waited for baby Malia to come on her own time—when she was ready.

The point I want to make is this: God is good. No matter what news you may get about your baby, God is there with you. At first, the news may be devastating to you, but the Lord always has a plan. We may never know exactly what His plans are, but we do know that Jesus said, "I will never abandon you or leave you" (Hebrews 13:5, *GOD'S WORD*).

After God turned Malia to the head-down position, the pre-labor contractions grew stronger. You may be feeling what's often called Braxton Hicks contractions, or false labor, this week, as I did. If so, don't be alarmed as the contractions work to help prepare your body for birth.

How can you tell if it's the real thing or just pre-labor contractions? Here are some tips to distinguish the two:

- True labor contractions grow stronger and don't go away if you lie down or sit in a warm, relaxing tub.
- True contractions grow closer together and last longer.
- Braxton Hicks tend to be felt only in front and not all over.
- Walking has no effect on Braxton Hicks, whereas walking makes true contractions stronger.
- The cervix doesn't change with Braxton Hicks, whereas the cervix opens and thins with true labor.

In general, if you have contractions less than 12 minutes apart during week 37 or earlier, it might be a sign of preterm labor, and you should contact your physician or midwife. If you're past 37 weeks, you usually won't need to contact your care provider until the contractions last about 60 seconds each and are 5 minutes apart. But follow the instructions you've been given by your own doctor. Each woman is unique, and your own doctor knows your individual pregnancy history and will have instructions for when to call.

A MOTHER'S PRAYER FOR WEEK 37

Dear Lord, I pray for my baby this week. I pray that You will turn my baby's head down in the direction You want her to be. If for some reason the baby shouldn't turn, such as if the cord is wrapped around her neck, then I pray that You take care of this situation too.

God, You are Almighty and know everything that is going on with my body and my baby. You know the exact minute that my baby is coming.

Lord, this has been a week of learning to trust in You. Your ways are higher than our ways, and Your thoughts are higher than ours. I place myself and my baby in Your hands and trust in You.

I know I can do all things You require of me, with Your help. You are here with me now, every minute of the day and night. I know You will take care of my baby. Lord, I receive Your peace and I place my trust in You. In Jesus' almighty name. Amen.

Scriptures for Thought and Meditation

Be strong and courageous. Don't be terrified or afraid. For it is the LORD your God who goes with you; He will not leave you or forsake you. He will be with you. Do not be afraid or discouraged.
DEUTERONOMY 31:6,8

Cast all your anxiety on him because he cares for you.
1 PETER 5:7, *NIV*

My Journal

My feelings about natural childbirth and a Cesarean birth:

_____
_____
_____
_____
_____
_____
_____
_____
_____
_____
_____

What I have done with all of my anxiety:

_____

_____

_____

_____

_____

_____

_____

_____

_____

_____

_____

_____

What Matthew 11:29-30 says to me:

_____

_____

_____

_____

_____

_____

_____

_____

_____

_____

_____

38

God Knows What You're Going Through

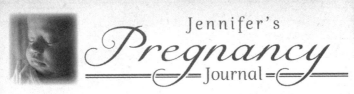

Jennifer's *Pregnancy* Journal

My doctor said the baby might come early, so I thought this was the week. My work schedule has lightened up a bit and, just in case, I warned my clients that I may have to cancel their fitness session if I went into labor. Of course they all understood.

Everywhere I go, people ask when my baby is coming, and I tell them, "Hopefully, today!" Then they congratulate me and wish me luck.

Every day I talk to the baby and encourage him, "Come out and meet the world."

But it hasn't happened yet. God is teaching me patience.

I went to get my new driver's license and had to wait more than two hours, so I left and came back and then discovered I'd missed my number. So I sat there another hour and finally got my picture taken. What a pain. At least when I look at my photo, I know I'm not alone in it.

We also had our neighborhood barbeque this week. We're blessed to have such great friends. We all watch out for each other, and we get to-gether a couple times a year. The cookout was a lot of fun. They even bought me a cake with a stork on it. They are so thoughtful.

Your baby could come any time now, or she could take a few more weeks to grow bigger and have her lungs develop just a bit more. God knows the exact minute your baby will be born, so try to be pa-tient, double-check your list to make sure everything is ready, and then trust in Him. This week, I have another pregnancy story to share with you—one that is unlike any of the others in this book, because it starts off with a misunderstanding.

It's about a young woman who was engaged to be married and then discovered she was pregnant. Needless to say, this came as a complete surprise.

She knew she had to tell her fiancé, and when she did . . . well, let's just say it didn't go very well. Although he truly loved her, he became angry and upset at this news.

He said, "This baby is not mine! I know it can't be mine."

She didn't argue because she knew it was true. She and her fiancé had not slept together; they had agreed to wait until they got married. So the fiancé said he was breaking off the engagement, and with a broken heart, he left her, utterly depressed. At this point, a lot of guys would have hit the bottle and gotten drunk to deal with the situation, but he was a decent guy, so he just went home to bed.

Now the young woman had to do something, because in her culture being an unmarried mother was not acceptable. It was considered unforgivable. In fact, a woman could even receive the death penalty for becoming pregnant by someone who was not her husband.

But now here's something surprising. This woman did not try to hide her pregnancy. She packed a bag and went straight to visit her cousin who lived in a neighboring town—who happened to be married to the highest religious leader in the country, the very one who could issue the order to have her put to death.

She wasn't completely sure how her cousin would react, because her cousin had been wanting to get pregnant herself for many years, and had not been able to conceive and was now past menopause. But still, the young, pregnant woman was hoping that her cousin would take her in and guard her life. She figured that her cousin was married to the man who had the authority to do that, and she was hoping her cousin would be able to persuade him, because they were family.

So the pregnant woman sped to her cousin's place, and when she got to the door, she called out, "Hello!"

At that very moment, the cousin, a woman named Elizabeth—who unbeknownst to the young expectant mom had received a miracle from God and was now six months pregnant herself—exclaimed in a loud voice, "You are the most blessed of women, and your child will be blessed!"

This seemed like a strange thing to say when the younger woman hadn't even told her cousin that she was pregnant; but the Holy Spirit had come upon cousin Elizabeth, and she spoke a word of prophecy.

Elizabeth went on to say, "How could this happen to me, that the mother of my Lord should come to me? For you see, when the sound of your greeting reached my ears, the baby leaped for joy inside me!"

And you know the rest of this story. The young woman named Mary ended up staying with Elizabeth and her husband, Zechariah, the high priest, for three months, and then she returned safely to her home. In the meantime, the depressed fiancé had a special visitor himself. The angel of the Lord showed up in his bedroom, woke him from his sleep and informed him that his beloved fiancée, Mary, had not been unfaithful, but that she'd been chosen by God to be the mother of Jesus, the long-awaited Messiah, the Savior of the world.

Can you imagine how stunned Joseph must have been? I mean, no woman he'd ever heard of had become pregnant while being a virgin. You can't really blame the guy for breaking up with Mary when he thought she was playing around while they were engaged. So anyway, Joseph got totally psyched and felt honored that he would be the stepfather to Jesus; and then he and Mary went through with their plans and had the wedding. The Bible doesn't give us any details about the wedding ceremony, but I suspect they were both deliriously happy about their future together.

But there was no honeymoon—not until after Jesus was born. So the prophecy was fulfilled that the Savior would be born of a virgin.

It's a remarkable, beautiful story. To think that God would design a plan to rescue us from our own sinful doom through a virgin birth is beyond amazing. And I love the part about cousin Elizabeth also conceiving when it was humanly impossible. She gave birth to John, commonly called John the Baptist, because he baptized Jesus in water at the start of Jesus' ministry.

I just had to include this story—the most miraculous of all pregnancy and birth stories—as you pray through your pregnancy. Below are the Scriptures that tell the story in a more elegant style.

This week, we pray a prayer of thanksgiving to God for His wonderful Son.

A MOTHER'S PRAYER FOR WEEK 38

Dear Lord God, I thank You from the bottom of my heart for giving us Your Son, Jesus. It's such an amazing story, what You did for us. I pray You will give me courage and faith like Mary had.

And, Lord, only You know the exact minute my baby will be born. Please help me to be patient and get through this time of waiting. I am so anxious to see and hold my baby that I can barely wait another day. Please be close to me and surround me with Your love and presence at the birth. Help the labor go smoothly and the birth to go just right.

Thank You, Lord, for all You have done to provide us with a way to communicate with You. Thank You for salvation and for Your great love. Thank You for my baby.

In Jesus' name. Amen.

Scriptures for Thought and Meditation

Luke 1–2
(These chapters tell the story of Jesus' birth, written by Luke.)

Matthew 1:18-24
(These verses give more perspective on Jesus' birth, written by Matthew.)

My Journal

What I love most about the story of Jesus' birth:

_____
_____
_____
_____

_____

_____

_____

_____

_____

_____

_____

_____

How Jesus' birth has been celebrated in my family (any traditions?):

_____

_____

_____

_____

_____

_____

_____

_____

_____

_____

_____

Ideas and plans for celebrating Jesus' birth with my child/children:

_____

_____

_____

_____

_____

_____

_____

_____

_____

_____

_____

39

One Week to Go!

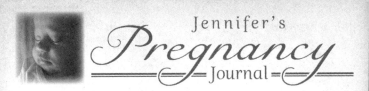

Jennifer's
Pregnancy
Journal

I called Janet, my doula, today right after I had another ultrasound. It's March 13, and I wanted her to know that the baby's head was still down. Praise the Lord!

I'd been up two nights in a row having contractions all night, and Janet says there's been some progress. Hopefully, it won't be long now. Even if those contractions weren't actual labor, at least they are conditioning my uterus for labor. Having had a baby before, I now know which contractions to pay close attention to and which ones to let pass by. These were not it, but I am ready for this baby to come, even though my official due date isn't until Easter Sunday, March 23. I would like my baby born on Easter—what a great day to have a baby, the day Jesus rose again!

One week to go! If you're like me, you are *so ready* for your baby to be born. Some babies will arrive early. That's what happened with my second baby, Malia. So fast-forward two-and-a-half years, and here is her story. As you recall from chapter 37, God miraculously turned her from being in the breech position to head-down after my pastor prayed, two weeks before her birth.

Micah and I were in the kitchen making breakfast, and I was still having contractions that began during the night. During every contraction I squatted down and did my deep-breathing exercises, and when I did, little Micah walked over to me, gently rubbed my back and said, "I love you, Mom." It was so sweet I wanted to cry. And it made the contractions go away a lot quicker—or so it seemed.

Dan arrived home from work that afternoon, took one look at me and knew that today was the day. We said a family prayer together, knowing that our family would soon be a foursome. We prayed for a quick, safe, easy birth and that the right person would be available to watch Micah while I was in labor. We have no family in town and our church friends were in Mexico on a mission trip. We'd made preliminary plans for my friend Claire to watch him, but it's just hard to schedule when you don't know exactly when the baby's coming. And especially now when I was going into labor early.

We drove to my doctor's office for my 2:15 appointment, and she gave us good news. Praise God, the baby was on the way! My contractions were now 10 minutes apart, and my doctor said to go home, get my bag and then head for the hospital.

We arrived at the hospital at 5:15 P.M. We settled into our room in "The Starting Place," a triage area. During the car ride the contractions increased to about five minutes apart and were a 5 out of 6 on the intensity scale.

At the hospital the contractions progressed and my baby was sitting low, fully engaged. At 5:55 P.M., the monitor said the contractions were just three minutes apart. At 6:20 P.M., Dan, Micah and Janet were ready for dinner, so we all trooped off toward the cafeteria. Dan and Micah went ahead; Janet and I trailed behind with me stopping for each contraction. There I was, wearing shorts and two gowns—one to cover the front and one to cover the back—and tennis shoes. What a sight!

I didn't want to eat, but the other three did. At 6:40 P.M., the gang was enjoying their food, and I felt something weird. I thought my water bag broke, because all of a sudden my contractions progressed quickly to about two minutes apart.

I said, "We need to go upstairs, *NOW!* This baby's coming."

Upstairs, I settled in to the "real" Labor and Delivery. The baby's heartbeat was doing great and there were absolutely *no* signs of distress. *Hallelujah!* Within what seemed like minutes of our arriving upstairs, and shortly after the water bag broke again, I said, "I feel like I want to push."

My friend Claire showed up just in time to take care of Micah and relieve my doula of that duty. Janet and Micah were down the hall looking at the babies in the nursery when Claire arrived. Janet literally sprinted back to my room, and she traded places with Dan, who'd been doing a great job of coaching me up to that point.

I pushed for about 10 minutes through two or three contractions—and then at exactly 9:32 P.M., on March 19, 2008, my little girl, Malia Grace, was here. Praise God!

The Lord was with me through the entire time, and He answered my prayers for a smooth, fast delivery.

She was 6 pounds, 8.8 ounces, 18-1/2 inches long and the picture of perfect health. I got to hold my little baby daughter snugly on my chest. What an indescribable experience it was to meet my daughter and cuddle her close to me. My heart was filled with love. God truly had grace on me that day, and that's why Malia's middle name is Grace.

Dan cried with joy when he saw his baby daughter. "It's a girl, my little girl," he said. I think we all cried then, overcome with happiness and gratitude to the Lord. God is so good!

Micah is so sweet with his new little sister, just as I expected him to be. I'd been praying daily throughout my pregnancy that he would be a good big brother and that they would be best friends—and God heard and answered my prayers.

This week is a week to praise God. The more you praise Him, the more He will shower His blessing down upon you. Instead of thinking how scared you are of labor or fearing how much pain you might have, thank God for giving you this wonderful experience and tell Him you can't wait to meet your baby. He will bless you beyond measure. He has great blessings in store for you. Let's just praise Him and give Him all of the glory.

A Mother's Prayer for Week 39

Dear Lord, I come to this week with praise in my heart. I know that in Nehemiah it says that Your gracious hand is upon me. I know You will bless this delivery, Lord. I know that my labor will be manageable and You will be with me the whole time. Please take away any fear that I may have, and help this baby to come quickly and safely.

You are a great and powerful God. I know that if I praise You, You will rain down Your blessings from above. I believe that You are the Alpha and the Omega, the Beginning and the End. This is a new beginning for my baby, for our family. We praise You for this wonderful gift. Thank You. In Jesus' name. Amen.

Scriptures for Thought and Meditation

The LORD is my strength and my song; He has become my salvation. This is my God, and I will praise Him.
EXODUS 15:2

To You, my strength, I sing praises, because God is my stronghold—my faithful God.
PSALM 59:17

My Journal

I would like to praise God for giving me peace about my labor and delivery. My favorite Scripture verse to read and meditate on whenever I feel afraid is:

_____

_____

_____

_____

_____

_____

The first three things I plan to do when we get home with our new baby:

_____

_____

_____

_____

_____

_____

40

Welcome, Baby!

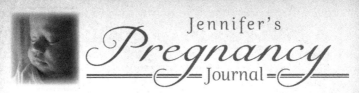

Jennifer's *Pregnancy* Journal

I kept my calendar open this week for the baby to come. My due date was on Monday and now it's Friday. Still there's no sign of the baby. What's going on? I feel like I'm going to be pregnant FOREVER.

He was supposed to be here on the twenty-fifth of July or sooner, according to the doctors. I keep walking on the trails behind my house, trying to help this baby along. I tried some completely safe natural remedies that people swear by, like eating spicy foods, but all that did was make my tummy upset!

I called Betty, my massage lady, to come over and try to help this baby along, too, but that didn't work either. It did make me relax though, and she assured me that the baby would be here in God's time, not ours. I know she's right. Every pregnancy is different, every labor is different and every birth is different. God knows what He is doing.

As you're getting ready to welcome your new baby into your home, I'd like to share with you some tips on having an easier labor and delivery. Every woman is unique, so pick and choose the ones you like—and always follow your doctor's advice.

Ten Tips for Having a Good Labor and Delivery Experience

1. *Let go of fear.* Stress, tension and fear make pain worse, so there's no sense in holding on to those negative emotions.

Trust is a choice. We can choose to say no to worry and yes to placing our trust in the Lord. This week is a good time to meditate on Scriptures like Proverbs 3:5-6.

2. *Concentrate on the positive.* "I am getting better at relaxing." "Labor is a natural process." "I can do this." Speaking positive affirmations goes a long way toward having a better birth experience.

3. *Have a good coach.* Having the support of someone who helps you relax, stay positive and do the breathing techniques is one of the best secrets for having a good labor experience.

4. *Use the breathing techniques.* Practice the breathing techniques you learned in childbirth class. They really do help.

5. *Be mobile.* Many women find they are better able to deal with contractions by pacing around rather than lying down, as this gives them a greater sense of being in control. Movement also helps relax the muscles and can prevent you from feeling too tense. I walked the halls in the hospital in my gowns to try to get the baby moving, and the contractions weren't nearly as intense as when I was lying down.

6. *Try warm water.* Some women prefer to sit in a warm tub or to take a shower during labor.

7. *Use massage therapy.* Have your husband or coach provide massage therapy with a firm touch. You can use almond oil or baby oil. I know I wouldn't have made it through the 30-plus hours of natural labor if it weren't for Janet, my doula, massaging my back during each contraction.

8. *Try squatting down, sitting up slightly, or another position.* For me, squatting during contractions made me feel better.

9. *Listen to music.* God gave us music to lift us up. God dwells in the praises of His people, so worship music brings the Holy Spirit into the room.

10. *Have prayer support.* Make a list of people who will agree to pray for you while you're in labor and delivery.

After Your Baby Comes

Up to now, you've been praying for your unborn baby, and very soon that changes. You will be praying for your son or daughter. Since you've built a good habit of praying for the past nine months, you're in a good position to continue your intercessory prayer ministry for your child. I believe that a mother's job of praying for her children never ends—at least not on this side of heaven.

Thank you for remaining faithful to prayer this far. If you believe in the message of this book, I would greatly appreciate it if you'd recommend it to other moms-to-be. Now, let's pray for God's help with your labor and delivery.

A MOTHER'S PRAYER FOR WEEK 40

Dear Lord,

This week is my due date. I thank You for helping me make it to full term in my pregnancy. I am looking forward to welcoming my baby into our home. Lord, please help my baby come at just the right time. Bless my labor and delivery. Give the medical staff wisdom to make all the right decisions. Help me be strong during delivery. Help me trust in You. I pray that Your sweet presence would fill the room with joy as I deliver the baby and we welcome him into this world.

Lord, I know You are a good God, and I choose to put my trust in You. Be with me now and every moment of the day. Let me be aware of Your presence with me. Reveal Yourself more to me so I can know You and love You more.

Thank You, Lord. In Jesus' name. Amen.

Scriptures for Thought and Meditation

Be still before the LORD and wait patiently for him.
PSALM 37:7, NIV

*From ancient times no one has heard, no one has listened, no eye has seen
any God except You, who acts on behalf of the one who waits for Him.*
ISAIAH 64:4

My Journal

My due date is:

_____
_____
_____
_____
_____
_____

My baby arrived on:

_____
_____
_____
_____
_____
_____

My "Welcome, Baby" message is (sign and date it):

_____
_____
_____
_____
_____
_____

41

Your Baby Might Be Late!

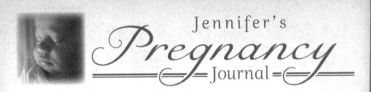

Jennifer's

Pregnancy
Journal

It's week 41, and I can hardly hold back the tears. He's never coming out!

I was convinced I would have my baby early, well before the due date. So when my due date came and went, it was very frustrating. I couldn't believe it! I was in shock, but more than that, I was so overly ready that I didn't have much to do in those last two weeks except wait and wait and wait.

Each minute of each day it was so hard to wait. I was so used to making goals for myself and then setting out to achieve them, one by one. This was a goal also, in a way, but one that I didn't have as much control over.

As I made my video journal on my due date, I commented about how I was supposed to have had my baby by now. Then, when I did the video a week later, I actually just burst into tears—hardly able to comprehend why I hadn't given birth already!

My due date was July 25, 2005, but the day came and went with no baby. The same thing happened the next day and the next, until the calendar turned to August.

August 1 nothing. August 2, nothing. And then the afternoon of August 3, contractions began—and continued all day and all night. Squatting seemed to be the best position for me, but after 24 hours of squatting and handling contractions, I was very tired. Fortunately, I was able to sleep for a few hours as contractions subsided.

At four o'clock the next day, I called Janet, my doula, to let her know. Dan was extremely comforting in wanting to do whatever he could to help. But I was pretty much handling them on my own and wanted to have him sleep instead. I figured I'd really need him later.

I think it was about 3:00 A.M. when I called Janet again, and God bless her for coming over in the middle of the night. Janet suggested I get in the tub for a while, in hopes of being able to catch up on some sleep. She stayed by my side for a long time, and then when she noticed that I was sleeping a bit between contractions, she moved to the bed, about 20 feet away.

Dan came upstairs at one point to check on us. He was much more interested in heading for the hospital than either Janet or I. We convinced him to go back to sleep, promising to call the doctor's office in the morning. I figured I would maybe go in *there* to have my cervix checked (rather than the hospital). I didn't want to go to the hospital just to be sent home again since it was so far away—a 30- to 40-minute drive each way.

When I called the doctor's office, they said something about me not *possibly* being in labor because I was interested in brushing my teeth and drying my hair (I had been in the tub half the night) before going in to the office. Nevertheless, we set an appointment, and off Janet and I went at about 8:30 A.M. We convinced Dan to head out to work, with a promise to call him if anything really changed. After all, this had been going on pretty much for two days already!

Emmy, my nurse, said, "You're dilated three to four centimeters."

I thought that was fantastic news. I said, "Praise God! At least these contractions are *doing* something!"

Emmy said, "I want you to check into the hospital by noon." But I had a different idea.

I was hungry, so we all ate lunch together back at home—with me standing up to lean forward, or squatting, during every contraction, and then Dan prayed for God's help and strength and we set off for the hospital to get there by two o'clock.

I did *not* enjoy the trip to the hospital, but then again, it wasn't as bad as I'd expected. The contractions were actually not as strong in the car—maybe it was the change of scenery.

I sat in the back seat per Janet's suggestion. Whenever a contraction came, I put one leg up on the seat, the other on the floor, and held on to the baby's car seat. I must have been *quite* a sight, and I remember wanting to wave at the people driving by who were gawking at me!

We arrived at St. Joseph's hospital in downtown Denver, and I hoisted myself out of the car. My water bag promptly broke all over the parking lot. Dan was so happy it didn't happen in the car!

However, when we got up to the maternity ward, they made the decision that my water bag had *not* broken. Imagine *that!* Obviously, *they* weren't in the parking lot when it happened.

I refused to let them check my cervix because I didn't want to risk introducing an infection since I *knew* my water bag had broken (even then they couldn't get any of their tests to "prove" it).

I continued squatting through every contraction. Dan kept giving me water to drink and put on some soothing Hawaiian music in the background. Over and over, I begged him to not fall asleep. I needed him now! One thing about my husband is that he can sleep anywhere, *anytime!*

He promised he wouldn't—and he didn't.

I remember sitting on the birth ball for part of the time, but mostly it's kind of a blur. It was difficult, I know that much! I also remember pushing for about an hour. I was really feeling out of it at that point since I hadn't slept in three days and had been in labor for more than 30 hours with no medication whatsoever. And I can't lie—it hurt!

Then, at exactly 9:28 P.M., on August 5, 2005, my beautiful baby boy, Micah Kekoa Polimino, was born! Praise the Lord! God is so good!

I could never have imagined the overwhelming love I would experience for this child. This was my own little boy, a part of me. I would do anything to protect him. I love him more than I love my own life. And then the realization hit me.

This is how God feels about us! It's amazing to think that God sent His own beloved Son, Jesus, to die for us on the cross, just so we might be with Him in heaven. How could He make such a colossal sacrifice for us? I certainly don't feel worthy, but experiencing the love I have for my own little boy, I finally get it. God did what was necessary to save us from evil.

When your baby comes and you hold your child in your arms, you'll understand what I'm talking about. This is truly a gift from God. We women are so blessed we get to experience this miracle of giving birth. It's truly amazing!

A Mother's Prayer for Week 41

Dear Lord,

You know when this baby is ready, and I will praise Your name. I have been waiting for what seems like forever. I feel so uncomfortable and truly can't wait much longer to meet my baby. Please make it happen soon. I know You have a reason for this delay, maybe a miscalculation on the date or maybe my baby's lungs need to mature a bit longer. Whatever it may be, I trust in You, God, and praise Your mighty name.

Jesus, give me peace and rest during these last days before the baby arrives. Make this baby healthy and strong. Please bring the right people to help me deliver this baby. Please let me have this baby in the way I wish, and in the way that's best for my child, whether natural or C-section. You know what is right for me and my baby.

You are a great and wonderful God who has given me a beautiful gift: the gift of life. I praise Your name, Jesus. Amen.

Scriptures for Thought and Meditation

He will yet fill your mouth with laughter and your lips with a shout of joy.
JOB 8:21

The LORD is my strength and my shield; my heart trusts in him, and I am helped. My heart leaps for joy and I will give thanks to him in song.
PSALM 28:7, *NIV*

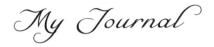

My Journal

Although this week may be difficult, some day you might look back and laugh. Or you might realize later that God taught you an important lesson during this time.

Record your thoughts on your day of delivery (for example: as you traveled to the hospital; as you were experiencing contractions; at the hospital when you knew the birth was imminent; what the coaching support of your husband or other birth coach meant to you; the first words out of your mouth when you held your baby for the first time, and so on).

_____

_____

_____

_____

_____

_____

_____

_____

_____

_____

_____

_____

_____

_____

_____

_____

_____

_____

_____

_____

_____

_____

_____

_____

When Something Goes Wrong

Carolyn Warren

Barbara is a mother of two, a beautiful woman who loves Jesus Christ more than anything else in her life, and who makes prayer a daily habit. When she and her husband learned they were expecting their third child, they were thrilled. As before, Barbara prayed and trusted God through her pregnancy.

January 13, baby David was born. At first, he looked perfect in every way, but that was not so. Along came subtle signs of something being wrong. Doctors didn't know what it was. The symptoms grew worse. And then, finally, the University of Washington Medical Center diagnosed David as having a progressive and incurable condition: Friedreich's ataxia, a rare type of muscular dystrophy. He'd been born with it. He would live to be about 18 to 20 years old, max.

Why, God? Why did it happen to this praying Christian family? Why David? Why my youngest brother? (Yes, Barbara is my mother.)

It didn't seem fair or right. The only conclusion we could come to was from the Scripture where Jesus told His disciples that no one was at fault for the man being born blind, but that it was to show the healing power of God. Jesus reached out and healed the blind man. So, as a family—and as a church—we prayed and interceded and believed for God to heal David.

Neither my parents nor David ever wavered in their faith.

God gave David 10 extra years beyond what the doctors predicted, but he died. Did God let us down? Did He let David down by not giving him a miraculous healing?

No, God did not let David down. He let him UP. David is now up in heaven, being rewarded for keeping his faith in the Lord Jesus

Christ in spite of what he went through. He's one of heaven's heroes. He's now having the most fantastic life ever, and he'll be there in his perfect heavenly body with the biggest grin on his face to greet me when I meet him there.

He'll say, "Hi, Sis, welcome to heaven!" And then perhaps he'll tell me that when he arrived in heaven, God asked him if he'd like Him to perform a miracle by healing him and raising him from the dead. And then David might tell me, "You know, Carolyn, I looked at the joy and beauty of heaven, and it took me one nanosecond to say, "No, thank You, God. Please don't send me back down there, not even in a healthy body. Let me stay. My family will all understand once they get here."

That right there is the key to the answer to all our questions of, "Why, God? Why my baby? Why did You let this happen?"

We may never understand now, but the answer will be clear once we get to heaven. I'm convinced that God has a different way of looking at things. What we consider to be a disaster on earth is not a disaster at all in the eternal perspective.

If you or someone you know has a baby born with Down's syndrome, like my dear, sweet Uncle Sherman, it's not a disaster. He or she is a beautiful soul who can love God with a pure, childlike faith and can spend forever enjoying all the delights of heaven. You call that a disaster? I don't think so. A disaster is a person with a perfect body and genius IQ who never chooses to make Jesus Christ his personal Lord and Savior.

There is so much more I could write about my brother David and other so-called disasters that happened, such as my grandma Edna's baby boy, John, who died shortly after being born. It was a heartbreak beyond compare, but you know what? John is up in heaven now having a long, beautiful life.

As I write briefly about these stories, tears come to my eyes. I can feel the heartache women experience when something goes wrong, things are not as planned. I would like to reach out to you and give you a hug and cry with you. Please feel free to write to Jennifer and me by going to the website www.PrayForYourBaby.com. We will stand with you in prayer. If you have a story to share, we'd love to read it, and we will personally reply to you.

And please remember, your story might end differently—God might miraculously heal your baby. A toddler named Joe drowned in a swimming pool, but God raised him up and he still lives today. He's my other uncle. A baby was born with a crooked foot, and as the pastor held the boy in his arms and prayed, the foot straightened out. That was my friend Cathy's baby, and the miracle baffled the doctors who were planning to do a series of bone breaks to straighten the foot.

But the important thing to remember is that God sees life differently from the way we do. God is love, and God has an eternal perspective that we don't have. As 1 Corinthians 13:12 says, "For now we see indistinctly" or in another translation, "through a glass darkly" (*KJV*). Our vision is obscured while we're here on earth. We can't answer all the whys.

We live in a fallen, sinful world, and not everything is going to be perfect here. The faith-filled, praying apostle Paul suffered many things—including unfair beatings and imprisonment, and an ailment he pleaded with God three times to take away, without success.

Jesus Christ Himself suffered while He was on this earth. If the perfect Son of God suffers, how can we expect our lives to contain no suffering? It's not possible.

So when something goes wrong, don't let it throw your faith for a loop. Continue praying, continue believing and continue loving God. Stand firm in your faith and claim one of my favorite Scriptures, Romans 8:35,37-39:

> Who can separate us from the love of Christ? Can affliction or anguish or persecution or famine or nakedness or danger or sword? No, in all these things we are more than victorious through Him who loved us. For I am persuaded that neither death nor life, nor angels nor rulers, nor things present, nor things to come, nor powers, nor height, nor depth, nor any other created thing will have the power to separate us from the love of God that is in Christ Jesus our Lord!

Jennifer's Testimony and Salvation Prayer

Jennifer Polimino

I grew up in a Christian home. I'm the second oldest of seven, and I have four brothers and two sisters. My parents decided they wanted us to live in a better place than Chicago, so when I was four, they moved to Hawaii. I'm glad they did because it is such a beautiful place to grow up. I realize that now that I'm gone, but not so much when I was younger.

My life changed when I was 12. I was molested by a group of four boys, and my attitude toward men changed forever. I figured that men only wanted one thing, and that one thing was the way to get their attention.

At 15, I had my first "boyfriend." He was 18, and I thought he was so cool on his way to college. Little did I know he had a bet going on with his friends to see how many girls he could "conquer" before he left. I was date raped.

Then I fell hard for a boy who I thought was the love of my life. We dated for a while and I then got pregnant, but we couldn't keep the baby—I was in the tenth grade! So I did the unthinkable at 16 and got an abortion. In my heart, I never wanted to do it, but I was only a teenager and all alone with this decision. I cried the whole time. I cut school, boarded a plane to Honolulu and was back home before dinner. My parents never even knew. I hated myself and didn't want to live, but I believed that if you took your own life, you would go to hell. This belief actually saved my life. After the abortion, I vowed never to have children. How could I be a good mother when I aborted my first child?

I struggled with this for years and years and went to counseling again and again in an attempt to "get over it." It never seemed to go away. As a result, I was in many unhealthy relationships. Then, thinking I should do it God's way, I got married after just six months of meeting someone. I divorced this abusive man and proceeded on to the next bad relationship.

This person talked me into doing things that I said I would never do. I had started competing in fitness competitions and soon the photographers wanted to take pictures of me. I was thrilled that someone thought I was pretty. But soon the photographers were asking me to do photos I now wish I hadn't done. At that point in my life, I was so far away from God that it didn't seem like a big deal; and I had people telling me that it was all right to do it. That led to other things I wish I hadn't done. Thank God He was still watching out for me all those years, even when I was so far away from Him.

God knew that the only way He was going to get my attention was through a man. That's when my husband entered the picture. In September 1999, I met Dan at a restaurant on a girls' night out. We had both been "dating" but wanted more. We decided we wanted this relationship to be according to God's plan. I quit my unhealthy night job, and I started going to church with him. We began planning our life together. But we had a long road ahead of us. The men in my past had destroyed so much of me. I still struggle with it on some days; but since my children have been born, God has healed me tremendously.

Our first year of marriage was very hard; we almost got divorced. We're both hardheaded people, and he had issues from his past too. But soon life took over and the bills started piling up. We both worked long hours and tried everything to make our business succeed, doing it our way and not God's. As we entered our fifth year of marriage, we decided that it was time to have a baby. I had put it off for a long time. I was so scared of losing my body and afraid that I wasn't going to be a good mother.

Financially, starting a family would be a strain on us, and I did not want a baby unless I could be a stay-at-home mother like my mom was. That would take away half of our income. In my heart, I knew that God would provide for our needs—and He always has. Some months have been really tight, but we still have a roof over our heads and food on the table.

Something happened when I became pregnant. Even though I was a Christian and had accepted Jesus as my Lord and Savior, I still didn't *know* Him. But during my first pregnancy, I grew closer to God than ever before. There was never a day that went by that I didn't pray for my baby. I prayed for health, joy and wisdom every day. Each week I researched the baby's development, and I prayed for that specific thing. And you know what? God answered every single prayer for my child. Micah Kekoa Polimino came into this world on August 5, 2005, and I have never been happier in my life. I used to say, "I'm never having kids, no way." Thank the Lord that He had different plans for me and has blessed me so much with this beautiful little soul. God answered every specific thing I asked for. Micah is a very healthy child. He was one of the happiest baby's in the world—he rarely cried. He started smiling, and I mean *real* smiles, at four weeks old. And God has blessed him with a tremendous memory. At 24 months he could recite the twenty-third psalm and the Lord's Prayer. Praise God! And he knows at least 15 Bible verses; and because of him, I know them too. I can honestly say that my children are the reason I am closer in my walk with God than ever before.

Every day, God is teaching me something about Himself through this little boy. He's teaching me about compassion and grace; about unconditional love and trust. And now the best thing is that Micah just became an older brother. Malia Grace came into our lives on March 19, 2008. She is as much of a blessing as her brother. I can see that the special prayers I've prayed for her are already coming to pass.

As you can see, it doesn't matter what you've done in your past. I'm not a perfect mother—far from it—but I do my best; and most importantly, I teach my kids about Jesus, our Lord and Savior.

If you feel like you want to be closer to God, too, it's very simple. All you have to do is ask the Lord Jesus to forgive you, and He will bury your sins in the deepest part of the ocean, never to be seen again. Isn't that a great word picture? Micah 7:19 says, "You will cast all our sins into the depths of the sea." And Hebrews 8:12 says, "For I will be merciful to their wrongdoing, and I will never again remember their sins."

God loves you no matter what you may have done. That's why He sent His Son, Jesus, to die on the cross for all our sins. Jesus paid the penalty for you and for me, and when you choose to believe and accept Him as your personal Savior and Lord of your life, you are born into the family of God.

John 3:16 says, "For God so loved the world in this way: He gave His One and Only Son, so that everyone who believes in Him will not perish but have eternal life." God loves you and wants to spend eternity with you.

God wants you to accept His gift of eternal salvation through Jesus Christ. Second Peter 3:9 says the Lord "is patient with you, not wanting any to perish, but all to come to repentance." God does not condemn you or me; He simply wants us to repent and change our ways.

God will forgive you and accept you. Romans 10:13 says, "For everyone who calls upon the name of the Lord will be saved."

First John 1:9 says, "If we confess our sins, He is faithful and righteous to forgive us our sins and to cleanse us from all unrighteousness."

If you haven't already done so and would like to ask Jesus to be your Lord and Savior, all you have to do is say this salvation prayer with me. Or if you would like to make a rededication to Jesus, you can pray this prayer again.

Salvation Prayer

*Dear Jesus, I believe You are the Son of God
and that You died for me on the cross so that I may live
with You in heaven forever. Please forgive me for
my sins and give me the gift of eternal life.
I want You to be part of my life. Please come into my heart today.
I want to know You and serve You always.
In Your name I pray, Jesus. Amen.*

Welcome to God's Family

If you prayed this prayer of salvation and you meant it from your heart, God has forgiven you of your mistakes of the past. Romans 10:9 reads, "If you confess with your mouth, 'Jesus is Lord,' and believe in your heart that God raised Him from the dead, you will be saved." That's His promise to you.

Our acceptance into the family of God is based on God's Word, not on what we feel. If you felt the presence of the Holy Spirit when you prayed, that's wonderful; but even if you felt nothing, you are accepted by Jesus Christ, because the Bible says so. God loves you. Luke 15:7,10 says all the angels in heaven rejoice when one person prays the prayer of salvation; and that means there is a celebration going on in heaven right now over YOU. As you read God's Word and worship Him, you will get to know Him more, and His love will become increasingly real to you.

Your next step as a new follower of Jesus is to read the Bible daily and find a good church to attend so you can grow in your faith. I recommend starting with the New Testament book of Mark, because it's a short book and it tells the story of Jesus. After that, you can read your way through the New Testament books. Save the Old Testament books, which were written to people before the birth of Christianity, until after you read the New Testament. And welcome to the family of God! We couldn't be more pleased!

Did you become a follower of Jesus today?
Please let me and
Carolyn know so we can pray for you. Go to
www.PrayForYourBaby.com and email us a note.

Are you already a follower of Jesus? You can also visit us at the above email address and let us know how you are doing and what prayer requests you may have.